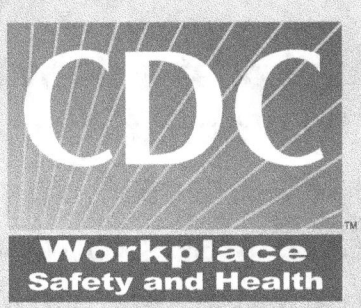

Evaluation of Chemical and Particle Exposures During Vehicle Fire Suppression Training

Kenneth W. Fent, PhD

Douglas E. Evans, PhD

James Couch, MS, CIH

Health Hazard Evaluation Report
HETA 2008-0241-3113
Miami Township Fire and Rescue
Yellow Springs, Ohio
July 2010

Department of Health and Human Services
Centers for Disease Control and Prevention

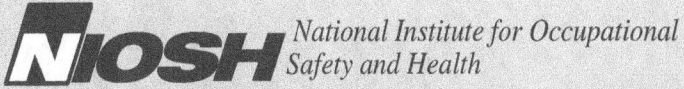
National Institute for Occupational Safety and Health

The employer shall post a copy of this report for a period of 30 calendar days at or near the workplace(s) of affected employees. The employer shall take steps to insure that the posted determinations are not altered, defaced, or covered by other material during such period. [37 FR 23640, November 7, 1972, as amended at 45 FR 2653, January 14, 1980].

CONTENTS

Abbreviations

$\mu g/m^3$	Micrograms per cubic meter
μm	Micrometers
$\mu m/cm^3$	Micrometers per cubic centimeters
$\mu m^2/cm^3$	Squared micrometers per cubic centimeters
ACGIH®	American Conference of Governmental Industrial Hygienists
cc/min	Cubic centimeters per minute
CFR	Code of Federal Regulations
cm	Centimeters
cm^3	Cubic centimeters
CO	Carbon monoxide
CO_2	Carbon dioxide
DBA	di-*n*-butylamine
EIC	Ethyl isocyanate
EPA	Environmental Protection Agency
ft/min	Feet per minute
HDI	Hexamethylene diisocyanate
IARC	International Agency for Research on Cancer
ICA	Isocyanic acid
IPDI	Isophorone diisocyanate
MDC	Minimum detectable concentration
MDI	Methylenediphenyl diisocyanate
mg/m^3	Milligrams per cubic meter
MIC	Methyl isocyanate
mm	Millimeters
mph	Miles per hour
MQC	Minimum quantifiable concentration
N/A	Not applicable
ND	Non-detectable
NIOSH	National Institute for Occupational Safety and Health
nm	Nanometers
OEL	Occupational exposure limit
OSHA	Occupational Safety and Health Administration
PAH	Polycyclic aromatic hydrocarbons
PBZ	Personal breathing zone
PEL	Permissible exposure limit

ABBREVIATIONS
(CONTINUED)

PHI	Phenyl isocyanate
PIC	Propyl isocyanate
PPE	Personal protective equipment
ppm	Parts per million
REL	Recommended exposure limit
SCBA	Self-contained breathing apparatus
STEL	Short term exposure limit
TD	Thermal desorption
TDI	Toluene diisocyanate
TLV®	Threshold limit value
TRIG	Total reactive isocyanate groups
TWA	Time-weighted average
USC	United States Code
VOC	Volatile organic compound
WEEL	Workplace environmental exposure level
XAD-2	Polystyrene/divinyl benzene based polymer

The National Institute for Occupational Safety and Health (NIOSH) received a request for a health hazard evaluation (HHE) from the Miami Township Fire and Rescue in Yellow Springs, Ohio. The request concerned chemical and particle exposures during vehicle fire suppression training.

What NIOSH Did on the First Evaluation

- We sampled the smoke from the engine and cabin fires from one vehicle on September 25, 2008. These samples were collected to identify the main chemicals in the smoke.

- We took personal breathing zone (PBZ) air samples on fire fighters. The samples were collected to look for volatile organic compounds, specific aromatic hydrocarbons, and acrylonitrile.

What NIOSH Found on the First Evaluation

- We found high levels of hazardous chemicals in the vehicle fire smoke. However, the PBZ air concentrations were below occupational exposure limits (OELs).

What NIOSH Did on the Second Evaluation

- We used the results of the first evaluation to tell us what to sample for in the second evaluation.

- We took PBZ air samples on fire fighters during the engine and cabin fires from three vehicles on July 14, 2009. The samples were collected to look for specific aromatic hydrocarbons, aldeyhydes, isocyanates, and carbon monoxide (CO).

- We sampled near the vehicle fires for the same chemicals, except CO.

- We sampled the particles produced during the fires to characterize their size and concentration.

What NIOSH Found on the Second Evaluation

- Most of the PBZ air concentrations were below OELs.

- Two of 15 PBZ concentrations of formaldehyde were above the NIOSH ceiling limit. If the fire fighters had not worn SCBAs some of them would have been overexposed to formaldehyde, a carcinogen and respiratory sensitizer.

- One CO concentration was just below its OEL. So, overexposures to CO could occur. CO can deprive the body of oxygen.

- Some isocyanate concentrations were just below the OEL during cabin fires. One sample collected near the vehicle fires measured isocyanates above the OEL. So, overexposures to isocyanates could occur during cabin fire suppression. Isocyanates are respiratory sensitizers.

- A large amount of small particles were generated during the fires. Small particles may be more harmful than large particles because they can go deeper into the lungs.

What Fire Chiefs Can Do

- Continue to enforce use of SCBAs during vehicle fire suppression. Include this practice in written policy.

- Attack fires from upwind positions; this will further reduce fire fighters' exposures.

- Park the motor pump apparatus upwind of the fire. Doing so will lower exposures to the motor pump operator, who usually does not wear an SCBA.

What Fire Fighters Can Do

- Put on your SCBA before attacking a vehicle fire. Keep the SCBA on until overhaul is complete.

- Stay upwind of diesel exhaust sources such as exhaust pipes. Diesel exhaust contains harmful substances.

- Talk to the fire chief about any health and safety concerns.

SUMMARY

NIOSH evaluated fire fighter exposures to chemicals and particles during vehicle fire suppression training. We found many different chemicals and high particle concentrations during the fires. According to our measurements, the potential exists for overexposure to formaldehyde, isocyanates, and CO. We recommend that fire fighters wear SCBAs until overhaul is completed. We also recommend that fire fighters stand away from diesel exhaust and park fire apparatus upwind of the fires.

In July 2008, NIOSH received a health hazard evaluation request from management at the Miami Township Fire and Rescue in Yellow Springs, Ohio. The request concerned potential inhalation exposures during vehicle fire suppression training. We conducted our first evaluation on September 25, 2008, to identify the main chemical constituents of engine and cabin fires during a training exercise involving one vehicle (two sampling events). We found high levels of various hazardous chemicals that helped us determine what to sample for on the second evaluation. During our second evaluation on July 14, 2009, we measured fire fighters' personal exposures to chemicals and particles during the engine and cabin fires for three vehicles (six sampling events). We conducted PBZ air sampling for aromatic hydrocarbons, aldehydes, CO, and isocyanates. In addition, we sampled for particles and other compounds near the fire fighters suppressing fires.

In both evaluations, most of the PBZ concentrations we measured were below STELs. However, 2 of 15 PBZ concentrations of formaldehyde exceeded the NIOSH ceiling limit of 0.12 mg/m^3. Although all the PBZ concentrations of isocyanates were below the STEL of 44 µg/m^3, using statistics, we calculated a 27% probability of overexposure to isocyanates during cabin fire suppression. Most real-time CO measurements were below the NIOSH ceiling limit of 200 ppm; however, one measurement (196 ppm) taken in the PBZ of the fire fighter performing backup was just below this ceiling limit. We measured increased particle number and mass concentrations during the vehicle fire knockdown, which persisted through the overhaul phase of the fire response.

Our findings indicate a potential for acute overexposure to formaldehyde, CO, and isocyanates during vehicle fire suppression. A potential for fine particle exposure can occur at any point during fire suppression operations. The intensity and duration of both the chemical and particle exposures depends on the wind speed and direction. Therefore, we recommend that fire fighters wear SCBAs until completing overhaul. We also recommend that fire fighters stand away from any diesel exhaust and park fire apparatus upwind of the fires. In addition, the motor pump operator should remain upwind of the diesel exhaust emissions from the fire apparatus because they could contain harmful substances.

Keywords: NAICS 922160 (Fire Protection), fire suppression, vehicle fire, car fire, fire fighter exposures, particles, isocyanates, formaldehyde

INTRODUCTION

On July 22, 2008, NIOSH received a health hazard evaluation request from the Miami Township Fire and Rescue in Yellow Springs, Ohio. The request concerned potential inhalation exposures during vehicle fire suppression training. In response to this request, we conducted evaluations on September 25, 2008, and July 14, 2009.

The Miami Township Fire and Rescue conducts vehicle fire suppression training two to three times per year. Fewer than 4% of its fire responses (~400 total runs per year) are to vehicle fires, which is below the national rate of 20% [Ahrens 2004]. Salvaged vehicles are used in the training exercises, which take place in abandoned parking lots. Vehicle fire suppression training has three phases: (1) startup—when the fire is ignited and allowed to build, (2) knockdown—when the fire is suppressed with water, and (3) overhaul—when the fire fighters search for and suppress residual flames or flare-ups. Figures 1–3 provide photographs from these phases. During both evaluations, vehicle engines and cabins were separately set on fire with flares and accelerated with gasoline. The fire fighters waited 2–5 minutes to let the fires build before knockdown with water. Knockdown took 1–3 minutes and was followed by 1–4 minutes of overhaul.

The fire fighters wore full turnout gear and SCBAs the entire time they fought the fires, including during overhaul. Miami Township Fire and Rescue has a comprehensive written respiratory protection program that adheres to the OSHA Respiratory Protection Standard [29 CFR 1910.134] requiring annual medical clearance; respirator fit testing; and training on the use, maintenance, and care of SCBAs.

On the first evaluation, the engine and cabin of a 1991 Dodge Dynasty sedan were set on fire. Most of the belts and the battery were missing, and the gas tank had been emptied; the cabin interior was relatively unaltered. On the second evaluation, the engines and cabins were set on fire for three vehicles: a 1994 Ford Aerostar minivan, a 1986 Toyota Corolla sedan, and a 1986 Toyota Celica coupe. The belts, fluids, batteries, cushions, and upholstery were present in each vehicle, but the gas tanks had been emptied.

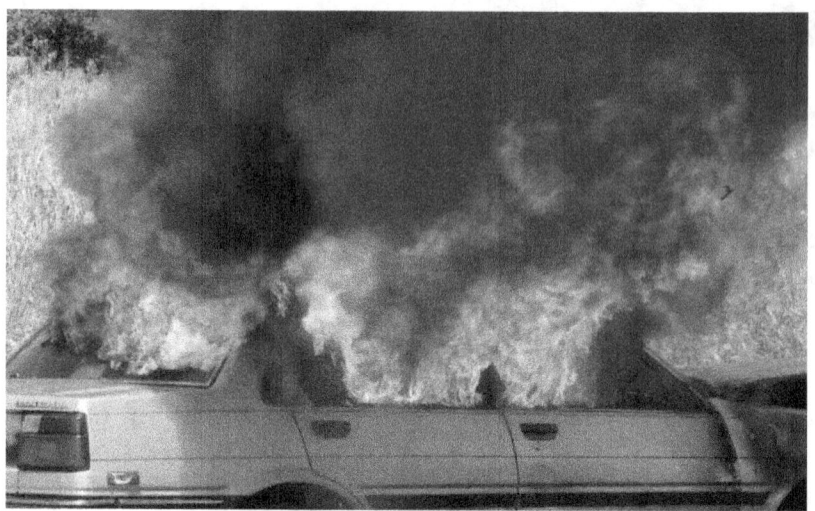

Figure 1. Startup phase of vehicle fire suppression training.

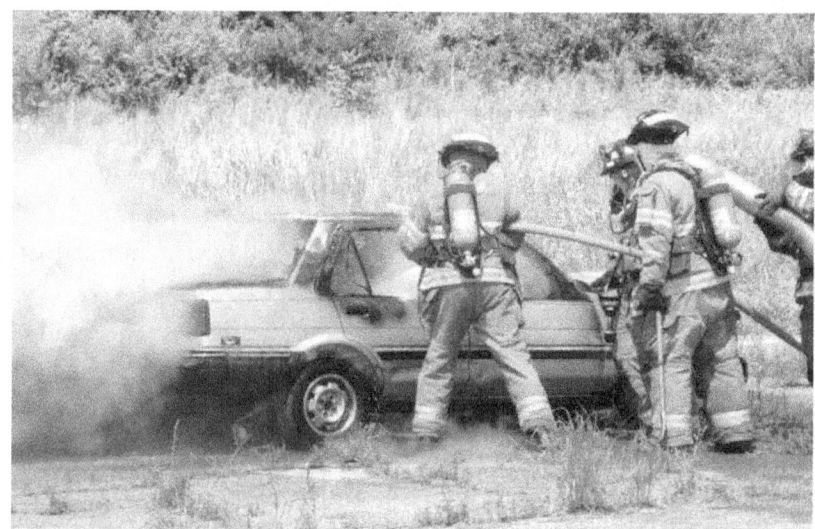

Figure 2. Knockdown phase of vehicle fire suppression training.

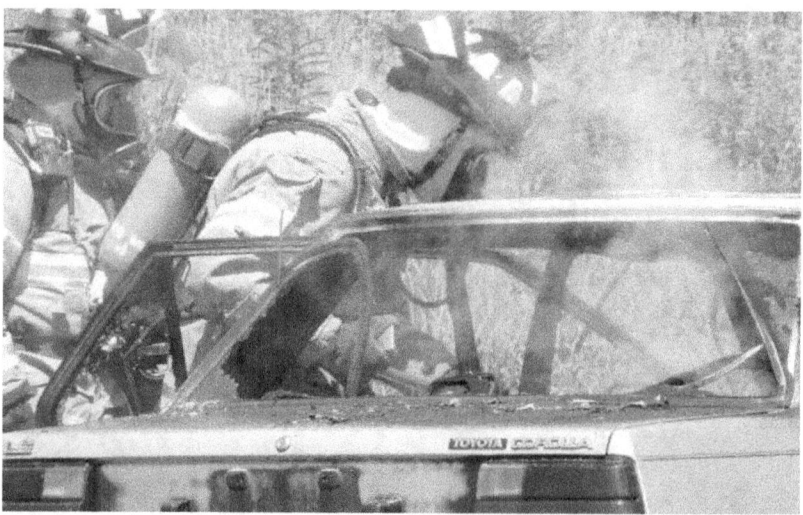

Figure 3. Overhaul phase of vehicle fire suppression training.

First Evaluation

Four fire fighters were involved in the suppression of the engine and cabin fires: a nozzle operator, a backup, a forcible entry, and an officer. The nozzle operator aimed the stream of water, backup assisted with holding the hose, forcible entry pried open doors or the hood to gain better access to the fires, and the officer managed the other fire fighters and assisted where needed.

We conducted PBZ air sampling and collected general area air samples of the smoke to identify chemicals emitted in the vehicle fires. A fire fighter in turnout gear and SCBA collected samples of the smoke from the engine and cabin fires. These samples were collected with 1-liter Summa canisters. The fire fighter collected the samples by holding the canisters in the smoke plume and opening the valve, which allowed the canister under vacuum to draw in 1 liter of the smoke (Figure 4). Six samples were collected in conjunction with startup, knockdown, and overhaul for each fire. Each sample of smoke was analyzed for VOCs. In addition, the four fire fighters suppressing the fires wore sampling trains containing TD tubes and charcoal tubes. The TD tubes identified the VOCs in the fire fighters' PBZs, while the charcoal tubes quantified the PBZ concentrations of the following aromatic hydrocarbons: benzene, toluene, styrene, and naphthalene. Charcoal tubes were also used to quantify acrylonitrile. We changed the sampling media between the engine and cabin fires. In addition, VOC samples (TD tubes and Summa canisters) were collected before any fires had been set to characterize the background levels of contaminants. More details on the sampling and analytical methods used during the first evaluation are provided in Appendix A.

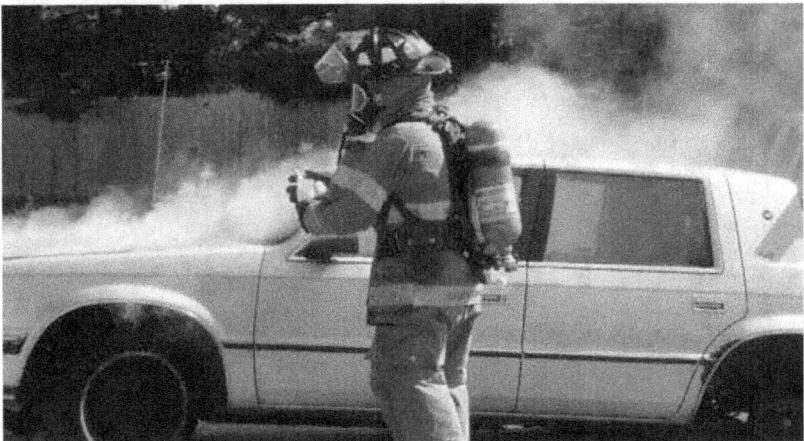

Figure 4. Fire fighter using Summa canisters to sample VOCs from a vehicle fire.

Second Evaluation

Five fire fighters were involved in suppressing the vehicle fires or assisting with sampling: a nozzle operator, a backup, an officer, a motor pump operator, and a duct holder (for particle sampling). The officer or backup performed forcible entry during this evaluation. Different fire fighters were involved with each vehicle burn; however, the same fire fighter operated the motor pump for all fires.

We conducted PBZ and general area air sampling for specific chemical compounds. Based on the results of the first evaluation, as well as an extensive literature review (see Appendix B for a summary of the literature review), we decided to sample for specific aromatic hydrocarbons, aldehydes, isocyanates, and CO. Aromatic hydrocarbons, aldehydes, and CO are common byproducts of organic material combustion. Isocyanates are used in the manufacture of polyurethane materials, and we speculated they may be released when combusting polyurethane foam used in automobile seat cushions.

Each of the five fire fighters wore three sampling trains. The sampling trains contained charcoal tubes, XAD-2 tubes, or denuders (Figure 5). Only the denuders were changed between the engine and cabin fires (except for the denuder worn by the motor pump operator, which was changed between each vehicle burned). The charcoal tubes were used to measure PBZ concentrations of the following aromatic hydrocarbons: benzene, ethyl benzene, naphthalene, styrene, toluene, and xylenes. The XAD-2 tubes were used to measure PBZ concentrations of the following aldehydes: formaldehyde and acrolein. The denuders were used to measure PBZ concentrations of the following isocyanates: TDI, MDI, HDI, PHI, MIC, EIC, PIC, IPDI, and ICA. The fire fighters also wore real-time monitors (GasAlert Extreme, BW Technologies Ltd., Calgary, Canada) to measure their PBZ concentrations of CO over time. More details on the sampling and analytical methods used during the second evaluation are provided in Appendix A.

General area air samples were set up around each vehicle to measure the same chemicals as for the PBZ sampling (except CO). The area air samples were approximately 25 feet west, south, and east of the vehicles. No area air samples were set up to the north because of a field with tall grasses. None of the area air samples

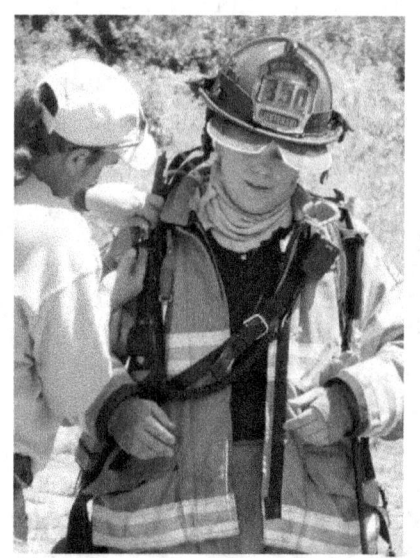

Figure 5. NIOSH investigator attaching a sampling pump to a fire fighter.

was changed between the engine and cabin fires. Table 1 provides an overview of the sampling scheme for the first and second evaluations, and Figure 6 provides a schematic of the second evaluation.

Table 1. Types and numbers of air samples collected during the first and second evaluations

Sampling media	Analytes	Method	Personal air sampling		Area air sampling (n)[†]	Smoke plume sampling (n)[†]
			N*	n[†]		
First evaluation						
Charcoal tubes[‡]	Acrylonitrile, benzene, naphthalene, styrene, and toluene	NIOSH 1501[¶]	4	8	N/A	N/A
TD tubes[‡]	Numerous VOCs (qualitative)	NIOSH 2549[¶]	4	8	N/A	N/A
Summa canister	75 VOCs (quantitative)	EPA TO-15**	N/A	N/A	N/A	6
Second evaluation						
Charcoal tubes	Benzene, ethyl benzene, naphthalene, styrene, toluene, and xylenes	NIOSH 1501[¶]	15	15	9	N/A
XAD-2 tubes	Formaldehyde and acrolein	NIOSH 2541[¶]	15	15	9	N/A
Denuders[§]	TDI, MDI, HDI, PHI, MIC, EIC, PIC, IPDI, ICA	[Marand et al. 2005]	15	27	9	N/A

* N = number of fire fighters sampled.
[†] n = number of samples collected. This number does not include blanks or background samples.
[‡] TD tubes and charcoal tubes (personal sampling) were changed between the engine and cabin fires during the first evaluation.
[§] Denuders were changed between the engine and cabin fires during the second evaluation for all fire fighters except the motor pump operator.
[¶] NIOSH Manual of Analytical Methods [NIOSH 2010]
** EPA Compendium of Methods for the Determination of Toxic Organic Compounds in Ambient Air [EPA 1999]

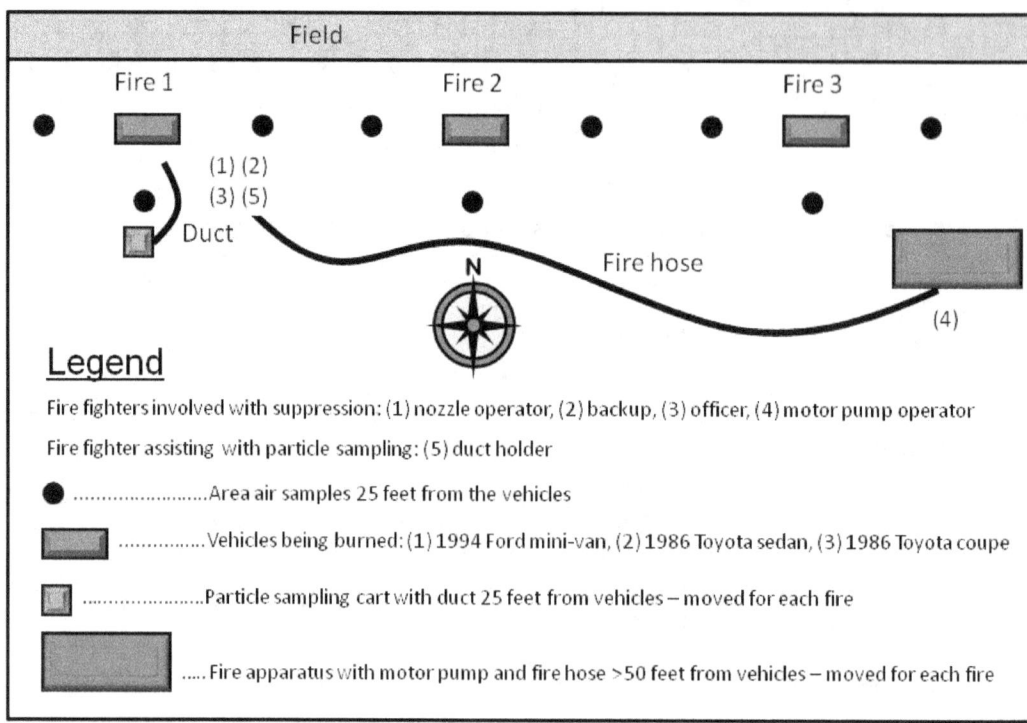

Field

Fire 1   Fire 2   Fire 3

(1) (2)
(3) (5)
Duct

N

Fire hose

(4)

Legend

Fire fighters involved with suppression: (1) nozzle operator, (2) backup, (3) officer, (4) motor pump operator

Fire fighter assisting with particle sampling: (5) duct holder

● ....Area air samples 25 feet from the vehicles

........................Vehicles being burned: (1) 1994 Ford mini-van, (2) 1986 Toyota sedan, (3) 1986 Toyota coupe

.......................Particle sampling cart with duct 25 feet from vehicles – moved for each fire

..... Fire apparatus with motor pump and fire hose >50 feet from vehicles – moved for each fire

Figure 6. Schematic of the second evaluation showing the location of the vehicle fires relative to the fire fighters, fire apparatus, and area samples.

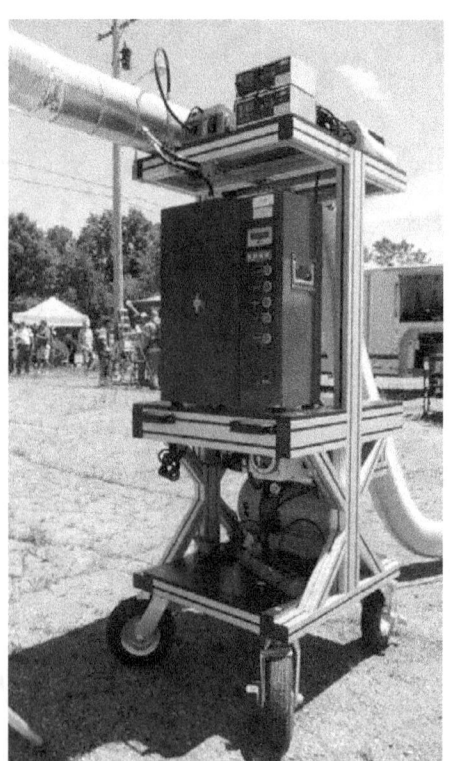

Figure 7. Photograph of the particle sampling platform housing multiple direct reading instruments.

Particles were sampled near fire fighters using 25 feet of flexible aluminum duct [Evans et al. 2010]. A blower unit downstream of the sampling platform drew smoke through the flexible duct. Multiple instruments then simultaneously and continuously monitored particles in the captured smoke. Particle metrics included number, active surface area, respirable mass, photoelectric response, and particle size distributions. A photograph of the particle sampling platform is provided in Figure 7. Appendix A provides more information on the particle sampling instruments and methodology.

In addition to chemical and particle sampling, we used a weather station to monitor weather conditions during the second evaluation (HOBO®, Onset Computer Corp., Bourne, Massachusetts). Air temperature, relative humidity, wind speed, and wind direction were recorded every minute. We also set up a thermal imaging camera (IR FlexCam Ti55, Fluke®, Everett, Washington) to capture images of the vehicle fires every 15 seconds to estimate the temperatures of the different phases of the fires. Finally, we recorded fire fighter activities with a digital camcorder (HDC-SD9P/PC, Panasonic®, Secaucus, New Jersey).

Because vehicle fires are generally suppressed quickly (< 15 minutes), STELs and ceiling limits are most appropriate for comparing the results of the personal air sampling rather than OELs that are usually based on 8-hour TWA exposures. Unless otherwise noted in this report, a STEL is a 15-minute TWA exposure that should not be exceeded at any time during a workday, and the ceiling limit is an exposure that should not be exceeded at any time. The NIOSH ceiling limit for CO is 200 ppm [NIOSH 2005]. The NIOSH and OSHA ceiling limits for acrylonitrile are 22 mg/m³ [NIOSH 2005]. The STELs and ceiling limits for the other chemicals we sampled are provided in Tables 2 and 3. Currently, no STELs or ceiling limits exist for PHI, MIC, EIC, PIC, or particles. More information on OELs is provided in Appendix C.

Table 2. STELs and ceiling limits* (mg/m³) for the aromatic hydrocarbons and aldehydes that were sampled during the second evaluation

	Benzene	Ethyl benzene	Naphthalene	Styrene	Toluene	Xylenes	Formaldehyde	Acrolein
NIOSH REL[†]	3.2	545	80	425	565	650	C 0.12	0.80
OSHA PEL[†]	16	N/A	N/A	C 850	C 1130	N/A	2.45	N/A
ACGIH TLV[‡]	8.0	545	80	170	N/A	650	C 0.37	C 0.23

* Ceiling limits denoted with the letter C.
[†] [NIOSH 2005]
[‡] [ACGIH 2009]

Table 3. STELs and ceiling limits* ($\mu g/m^3$) for the isocyanates that were sampled during the second evaluation

	TDI	MDI	HDI	IPDI	TRIG
NIOSH REL[†]	N/A	C 67	C 70	C 68	N/A
OSHA PEL[†]	C 68	C 67	N/A	N/A	N/A
ACGIH TLV[‡]	68	N/A	N/A	N/A	N/A
UK-HSE OEL[§]	N/A	N/A	N/A	N/A	70
Sweden OEL[¶]	N/A	N/A	N/A	N/A	44

* Ceiling limits denoted with the letter C.
[†] [NIOSH 2005]
[‡] [ACGIH 2009]
[§] [HSE 1999]
[¶] [Swedish National Board of Occupational Safety and Health 2000]

First Evaluation

The primary purpose of the first evaluation was to identify the main constituents in the vehicle fire smoke. Table 4 presents the concentrations of 10 VOCs for each phase of the engine and cabin fire suppressions as measured with Summa canisters. The compounds reported in Table 4 were selected based on their relative abundance in the sampled smoke and on potential toxicity. For an ordered list of the 15 most abundant VOCs and their respective concentrations for each phase of the engine and cabin fire suppression, see Tables D1 and D2 in Appendix D.

Table 4. Concentrations (mg/m^3) of 10 selected volatile organic compounds in the vehicle fire smoke measured during the first evaluation

Select compounds	Engine fire			Cabin fire		
	Start up	Knockdown	Overhaul	Start up	Knockdown	Overhaul
Benzene	5.2	1.6	11	60	1.4	0.38
1,3-Butadiene	2.3	0.40	4.8	6.8	0.25	0.05
Toluene	1.4	9.3	3.8	10	4.6	0.95
Naphthalene	1.4	0.93	1.2	10	0.60	0.17
Styrene	0.83	3.3	1.6	14	2.3	0.45
Acrolein	0.56	0.35	1.4	15	0.18	0.05
Methyl methacrylate	0.44	0.17	0.21	0.33	0.81	0.06
Acrylonitrile	0.32	0	0.77	27	0.38	0.07
Acetonitrile	0.28	0.12	0.70	14	0.12	0.03
Ethyl benzene	0.15	2.2	0.41	1.4	0.7	0.12

We identified the highest peaks in the gas chromatograms for the most concentrated VOC samples collected with TD tubes during the engine and cabin fire suppressions. Aliphatic hydrocarbons (pentane, chlorodecane, and various C_6 aliphatic hydrocarbons) and aromatic hydrocarbons (benzene, toluene, styrene, naphthalene, and xylenes) were elevated (compared to background samples) in the PBZs of the fire fighters during the suppression of the engine and cabin fires.

We also conducted PBZ air sampling for specific aromatic hydrocarbons during the first evaluation. Personal exposures are affected by wind speed and direction. The fire fighters at the Miami Township Fire and Rescue typically attack vehicle fires from an upwind position to minimize exposures and maximize visual perception. In this exercise, the fire fighters attacked the fires predominantly from the southeast direction. According to the National Weather Service [http://www.nws.noaa.gov], during this exercise, the wind was from the southwest (away from fire fighters attacking the fires) and averaged 14 mph, the temperature was 80°F, and the relative humidity was 30%.

Table 5 provides the PBZ concentrations of benzene and toluene measured during the cabin fire suppression. The MDCs and MQCs were calculated by dividing the respective analytical limits of detection and quantitation (mass units) by the minimum volume of air sampled. The MDCs and MQCs represent the smallest air concentrations that could have been detected (MDC) or quantified (MQC) based on the volume of air sampled. The PBZ concentrations of acrylonitrile, naphthalene, and styrene during the cabin fire suppression were ND (below their respective MDCs of 0.46, 2.3, and 0.11 mg/m³). The MDC for benzene was 0.09 mg/m³; for toluene it was 0.11 mg/m³. All PBZ concentrations measured during the engine fire were ND. (Note: The MDCs were the same for the cabin and engine fire suppressions.) All exposures were well below applicable STELs or ceiling limits. Concentrations between the MDC and MQC are listed in Table 5 and subsequent tables but are in parentheses to point out that there is more uncertainty associated with these values than with concentrations above the MQC.

Table 5. Personal breathing zone concentrations (mg/m³) of benzene and toluene measured during the cabin fire suppression on the first evaluation*

Job title	Sampling time (min)	Benzene	Toluene
Nozzle operator	22	(0.13)	(0.27)
Backup	22	ND	(0.12)
Forcible entry	23	ND	(0.12)
Officer	23	ND	(0.20)
MDC		0.09	0.11
MQC		0.34	0.41

* Values in parentheses represent concentrations below the MQC but above the MDC.

Second Evaluation

The goal of the second evaluation was to conduct a more thorough investigation of the chemical and particle hazards present during vehicle fire suppression by sampling for specific chemical compounds and characterizing particles in the air. Table 6 provides the PBZ concentrations of aromatic hydrocarbons and aldehydes measured during the second evaluation. The PBZ concentrations of naphthalene, styrene, and acrolein were ND (below the respective MDCs of 0.94, 4.7, and 0.16 mg/m³). Three samples of toluene and one sample of ethyl benzene had evidence of significant breakthrough, where the back section of the sampler collected >10% of the front section. These samples may have underestimated the actual air concentrations. Two of 15 PBZ samples measured formaldehyde above the NIOSH ceiling limit of 0.12 mg/m³.

Table 6. Personal breathing zone concentrations (mg/m³) of aromatic hydrocarbons and aldehydes measured during the second evaluation*

Job title	Fire	Sampling time (min)	Benzene	Ethyl benzene	Toluene	Xylene	Formaldehyde
Nozzle operator	1	55	(0.08)	ND	2.45	(0.12)[†]	ND
Backup	1	52	(0.10)	ND	(0.26)	ND	(0.04)
Officer	1	58	ND	ND	2.52[‡]	(0.10)[†]	ND
Motor pump operator	1	43	ND	ND	(0.09)[‡]	ND	ND
Duct holder	1	46	ND	ND	4.30[‡]	ND	ND
Nozzle operator	2	43	ND	ND	(0.14)	ND	(0.14)
Backup	2	40	ND	ND	(0.16)	ND	ND
Officer	2	46	ND	ND	(0.15)	ND	(0.05)[†]
Motor pump operator	2	48	ND	ND	0.69	ND	(0.06)
Duct holder	2	39	ND	(0.10)[‡]	ND	ND	ND
Nozzle operator	3	40	(0.08)	ND	(0.19)	ND	ND
Backup	3	43	ND	ND	(0.09)	ND	(0.06)
Officer	3	34	(0.14)	(0.15)	(0.44)	(0.25)	ND
Motor pump operator	3	43	ND	ND	ND	ND	ND
Duct holder	3	32	(0.16)	ND	(0.14)	ND	0.31
MDC			0.08	0.06	0.08	0.16	0.06
MQC			0.31	0.22	0.67	1.4	0.22

* Values in parentheses represent concentrations below the MQC but above the MDC.
[†] Calculated using a greater volume of air than that used to calculate the MDC.
[‡] Evidence of chemical breakthrough where the back section of the sampler collected >10% of the front section.

Table 7 presents the PBZ concentrations of isocyanates measured during the cabin fires on the second evaluation. Levels above the MDCs but below the MQCs were not reported by the analytical laboratory. Thus, ND represents concentrations below the respective MQCs. The PBZ concentrations of MDI, HDI, and IPDI were ND (below their respective MQCs of 1.8 µg/m³). The

RESULTS
(CONTINUED)

PBZ concentrations of MIC, EIC, and PIC were also ND (below their respective MQCs of 3.6 µg/m³).

TRIG is the concentration of all measurable isocyanate groups (N=C=O) in a sample of air. TRIG was calculated by multiplying the decimal percentage of isocyanate groups in the compound (the molecular weight of total isocyanate groups divided by the molecular weight of the compound) by the PBZ concentration (µg/m³) of that compound and adding the resultant values for all measureable isocyanate compounds. Because ICA has the greatest proportion of the isocyanate group (98%), it had the greatest influence on the concentration of TRIG. The detection limit for ICA was used to calculate the MQC for TRIG. In theory, the MQC for TRIG could be considerably less than 17.5 µg/m³.

Table 7. Personal breathing zone concentrations (µg/m³) of isocyanates measured during the cabin fire suppression on the second evaluation

Job title*	Fire	Sample time (min)	PHI	TDI	ICA	TRIG
Nozzle operator	1	15	3.20	1.54	16.2[†]	17.7
Backup	1	15	ND	ND	ND	ND
Officer	1	15	Sample excluded because of pump error			
Duct holder	1	16	ND	ND	ND	ND
Nozzle operator	2	14	ND	ND	19.7	19.2
Backup	2	14	ND	ND	ND	ND
Officer	2	14	ND	ND	ND	ND
Duct holder	2	14	ND	7.68	28.6	31.6
Nozzle operator	3	17	Sample excluded because of pump error			
Backup	3	17	ND	ND	ND	ND
Officer	3	17	ND	ND	ND	ND
Duct holder	3	18	ND	ND	ND	ND
MQC			3.6	1.8	17.9	17.5

* The motor pump operator wore the same denuder for both the engine and cabin fires; thus, his exposures (which were all non-detectable) are not reported.
[†] Calculated using a greater volume of air than that used to calculate the MQC.

For example, using the detection limit for TDI, we calculated an MQC of 0.86 µg/m³. However, we cannot assume that ND concentrations for TRIG would represent levels so far below 17.5 µg/m³, especially because ICA was the most abundant isocyanate species and was present in all samples with any detectable levels of isocyanates.

Because three samples of TRIG were just below the Swedish STEL of 44 µg/m³, we used statistical analysis to determine the likelihood of an overexposure (IHDataAnalyst V1.01, Exposure Assessment Solutions Inc., Morgantown, West Virginia). Maximum likelihood estimation was used for assigning values to the ND concentrations. According to this analysis, there is a 27% probability that the true 95th percentile for the PBZ concentrations of TRIG is above the Swedish STEL.

CO exposures for the fire fighters suppressing vehicle fires (nozzle operator, backup, and officer) are illustrated in Figures E1–E3 in Appendix E. None of the instantaneous measurements exceeded the NIOSH ceiling limit of 200 ppm. However, one measurement (196 ppm) collected in the PBZ of a fire fighter performing backup was just below the NIOSH ceiling limit. Therefore, the potential for overexposure to CO cannot be discounted.

The area sampling results are presented in Table D3 in Appendix D. Toluene, benzene, and TRIG were most frequently detected but the majority of the contaminants were ND. All of the concentrations were below applicable STELs except for one sample that measured TRIG concentrations above the Swedish STEL of 44 µg/m³.

Particle exposure was primarily influenced by the position of the fire fighters relative to the wind direction. Increased particle exposures were observed during knockdown and overhaul phases of fire suppression. Figures E4–E6 in Appendix E show time series data for particle measurements collected during the vehicle fires (engine fires followed by cabin fires). Figure E7 in Appendix E shows the particle number concentrations by different size ranges during the second evaluation. According to this figure, the ultrafine particles (< 0.1 µm in diameter) dominated the particle counts. Fifteen-minute TWA concentrations from each of the vehicle fires are presented in Table 8. Maximum transient concentrations of $1.2 \times 10^7/cm^3$ for particle number, 4700 µm²/cm³ for active surface area, and 170 mg/m³ for respirable particle mass were obtained throughout all six fires.

RESULTS
(CONTINUED)

Table 8. Particle measurements and CO concentrations for each vehicle fire expressed as 15-minute TWA concentrations

		Number (/cm^3)	Respirable mass (mg/m^3)	Active surface area (mm^2/cm^3)	Photoelectric response	CO (ppm)
Vehicle 1						
Engine	Mean	55,700	0.53	100	30	1.3
	Maximum	2,360,000	76	880	580	7.2
Cabin	Mean	88,500	0.13	110	10	0.6
	Maximum	1,443,000	12	560	60	1.7
Vehicle 2						
Engine	Mean	54,100	0.22	97	50	0.4
	Maximum	2,945,000	37	940	1000	1.5
Cabin	Mean	198,000	2.0	350	72	1.8
	Maximum	6,950,000	170	2600	1400	8.8
Vehicle 3						
Engine	Mean	52,600	0.33	80	8.0	0.4
	Maximum	1,380,000	51	680	97	1.6
Cabin	Mean	324,000	5.9	490	21	7.0
	Maximum	12,100,000	170	4700	340	62
Background*	Mean	20,400	0.007	14	3.0	0.1
	Maximum	24,700	0.011	20	5.0	0.3

* Background levels were determined by sampling the air prior to any of the vehicle fires.

A summary of the weather conditions during the second evaluation is presented in Table D4 in Appendix D. The wind direction during fire suppression varied, but was predominately southerly with an average speed of 2.6 mph. The fire fighters attacked the fires mostly from the south or southeast direction. Thus, the wind tended to blow away from the fire fighters. Nevertheless, we observed instances when the fire fighters encountered the smoke plume because the winds shifted or because the fire fighters changed positions to gain better access to the fire. The temperature increased slightly throughout the day (75°F–79°F), while the relative humidity remained steady (average of 33%). According to the thermal images (Figures E8–E11 in Appendix E), the cabin fires were hotter than the engine fires, and some metal parts of the vehicles remained hot (> 200°F) after knockdown. All but one fire exceeded 1000°F.

DISCUSSION

Vehicle fires, although suppressed quickly, can release hundreds of toxic chemicals into the air. Vehicle fire emissions include organic compounds (e.g., benzene, formaldehyde, hydrogen cyanide) and inorganic compounds (e.g., CO, sulfur dioxide, hydrogen chloride). Many of these compounds can be acutely toxic. Particles of various sizes and composition will also likely be produced and may cause health effects over short exposure periods. Even after the fire is extinguished, the release of potentially harmful chemicals and particles may continue. The purpose of our evaluation was to identify and quantify some of the potential acutely toxic chemical and particle hazards present in the air during vehicle fire suppression.

This evaluation has several limitations. Measuring all the harmful substances emitted in vehicle fires is not feasible. For example, although sulfur dioxide and hydrogen chloride can be acutely toxic and are likely to be present in vehicle fire smoke, we did not sample for them simply because we did not want to overburden the fire fighters with too many sampling pumps. The sampling media we used also have limitations. For example, charcoal tubes and XAD-2 tubes are designed primarily to measure gases and vapors. Thus, gases and vapors adsorbed to particles may not have been quantified with the sampling methods we used. In addition, vehicle fires are extremely hot. We observed flames that exceeded 1000°F and smoke that exceeded 300°F (see Figures E8 and E10 in Appendix E). Even after the initial knockdown, some metal parts of the vehicles exceeded 200°F (see Figures E9 and E11 in Appendix E). Elevated ambient temperatures (> 100°F) can cause a portion of aromatic hydrocarbons to pass through charcoal tubes. We saw evidence of this in that 3 of 15 PBZ samples of toluene had significant breakthrough (where the back section of the sampler collected > 10% of the front section). One sample of ethyl benzene also showed significant breakthrough. Therefore, the PBZ concentrations of aromatic hydrocarbons we reported may underestimate the true concentrations. Benzene, toluene, and ethyl benzene are the most volatile aromatic hydrocarbons we measured, and as such, would be most vulnerable to the effects of elevated ambient temperatures. This temperature effect is unlikely for XAD-2 or denuders because they are designed to derivatize chemicals during sample collection.

The duct and blower system utilized for the direct reading particle sampling had some limitations. Although the duct inlet was

DISCUSSION
(CONTINUED)

positioned close to the nozzle operator's shoulder by an assisting fire fighter, measurements should not be construed as actual PBZ concentrations for the nozzle operator or any other fire fighters. The movement of the nozzle operator and other fire fighters during fire suppression made exposure assessment challenging, particularly because particle concentration gradients close to burning vehicles were expected to be great. Nevertheless, the data presented here do provide some indication of particle concentration, duration of exposure, and size of particles anticipated during vehicle fire suppression. One further limitation of this evaluation was that compositional information of the emitted particles was not investigated.

Despite the limitations of this evaluation, we were able to characterize the fire fighter exposures to select aromatic hydrocarbons, aldehydes, isocyanates, CO, and particles. During the second evaluation, we found a potential for overexposure to formaldehyde and TRIG during vehicle fire suppression. Quantifiable levels of TRIG were only present in the air during the cabin fire suppressions. This finding makes sense given the large proportion of isocyanate-based foams that are used in the vehicle cabins. Exposures to CO were generally well below the NIOSH ceiling limit of 200 ppm. However, one measurement of CO (196 ppm) collected in the PBZ of the fire fighter performing backup during knockdown of an engine fire was just below the NIOSH ceiling limit (see Figure E1 in Appendix E). Thus, overexposure to CO is a possibility during vehicle fire suppression, especially when the fire fighters work close to the fires. All other PBZ concentrations were below applicable STELs or ceiling limits.

The chemical and particle levels we found were most likely influenced by the wind speed and direction. During the first evaluation, the wind was brisk (average of 14 mph) and blew away from 0he fire fighters. During the second evaluation, the wind was light (average of 2.6 mph) and blew in different directions (although predominantly away from the fire fighters). Therefore, we would expect greater exposures during the second evaluation than the first evaluation. Overall, the PBZ concentrations of toluene were higher during the second evaluation than the first evaluation. Concentrations of the other aromatic hydrocarbons could not be compared between evaluations because of the high percentage of ND concentrations.

DISCUSSION
(CONTINUED)

The area air sampling results from the second evaluation also provided evidence that contaminants were transported by the wind. Benzene, toluene, and TRIG were found in area samples from each fire. Area samples were not collected north of the vehicle fires. Because the winds were predominately southerly, this was probably the area where contaminant concentrations were the greatest. Nevertheless, one area sample collected west of the third vehicle fire measured TRIG concentrations that exceeded the Swedish STEL (44 $\mu g/m^3$). This finding provides additional evidence of a potential for overexposure to TRIG during vehicle fire suppression.

All the fire fighters in this evaluation except the motor pump operator wore SCBAs. The motor pump operator did not wear an SCBA because he was > 50 feet upwind from the fires and needed to easily communicate on the radio with the other fire fighters. The motor pump operator's PBZ concentrations, therefore, represent actual inhalation exposures. The motor pump operator was exposed to toluene and formaldehyde at concentrations below OELs. The source of these compounds could have been emissions from the vehicle fires or diesel exhaust from the fire apparatus [Ulfvarson et al. 1987; Smith et al. 2004; Mabilia et al. 2006]. For the other fire fighters, the PBZ concentrations we reported represent potential inhalation exposures due to the added protection of the SCBAs they wore. The OSHA assigned protection factor for a full facepiece SCBA used in positive pressure mode is 10,000 when fitted, maintained, and worn according to OSHA regulations [29 CFR 1910.134]; thus the inhalation exposures for the fire fighters who wore SCBAs are estimated to be 10,000 times lower than the PBZ concentrations we reported.

Fire fighters commonly do not wear SCBAs when responding to vehicle fires. According to an analysis by Austin et al. [2001], fire fighters in Montreal were estimated to wear SCBAs approximately 50% of the time at structural fires, but only 6% of the time at all fires (which included vehicle fires). Possible reasons for not wearing an SCBA during vehicle fires include the following: vehicle fires tend to be suppressed quickly (within a few minutes) and thus, exposures are assumed to be minimal, donning an SCBA takes time and is cumbersome to wear, and the belief that breathing air should be saved for more intense fires when it is really needed. Even when SCBAs are worn for vehicle fires, they may be removed during overhaul.

DISCUSSION
(CONTINUED)

Because fire fighters do not always wear SCBAs when responding to vehicle fires, the concentrations we measured indicate the potential for overexposure to some chemicals. In general, STELs and ceiling limits are intended to prevent acute health effects from short-term exposures. Short-term exposure to formaldehyde can cause eye and upper respiratory tract irritation [IPCS 2004]. Short-term exposure to isocyanates can irritate the respiratory tract and possibly lead to respiratory sensitization and occupational asthma [Chan-Yeung and Lam 1986]. Short-term exposure to CO can reduce the oxygen-carrying capacity of the blood, which may lead to asphyxiation or increase the risk for a cardiovascular event [IPCS 2007]. Chronic effects, such as cancer, generally require longer exposure periods. Cancer also has a latency period (10–30 years), which is the time between first exposure to a carcinogen and clinical recognition of the disease [Rugo 2004]. Of the chemicals we sampled, benzene and formaldehyde are considered carcinogenic to humans [IARC 1982a, 1982b, 1987, 2006]. Certain PAHs (e.g., benzo[a]pyrene and benz[a]anthracene), which may be produced during incomplete combustion of organic materials, are considered probably carcinogenic to humans [IARC 1983]. Although we did not quantify PAHs, the photoelectric aerosol sensor responds most strongly to particle emissions with surfaces enriched with PAH compounds [Siegmann et al. 1999]. The strong elevations in photoelectric response observed throughout sampling were most likely derived from particle surfaces with adsorbed PAHs. For more information on the potential health effects of the substances we sampled, see Appendix C.

Conclusions

Hundreds of organic and inorganic compounds in gaseous and particulate form may be released during vehicle fires and therefore may present a health hazard for fire fighters. We evaluated fire fighter exposures to chemicals and particles during vehicle fire suppression training. We identified the primary gases and vapors present in vehicle fire emissions and quantified the PBZ concentrations of some of these substances. Because vehicle fires are suppressed quickly, we compared the PBZ concentrations to applicable STELs and ceiling limits. We found a potential for overexposure to formaldehyde, TRIG, and CO. Although no STELs or ceiling limits exist for particle concentrations, we found increased concentrations of particle number, respirable particle mass, and active particle surface area during knockdown and overhaul of the vehicle fires.

Recommendations

Based on our findings, we recommend the actions listed below to create a more healthful workplace. We encourage Miami Township Fire and Rescue to use a labor-management health and safety committee or working group to discuss the recommendations in this report and develop an action plan. Because the vehicle fire suppression training took place in a parking lot, engineering controls (e.g , exhaust ventilation) are not feasible. Instead, fire fighters must rely on PPE and administrative controls for protection.

Personal Protective Equipment

Proper use of PPE requires a comprehensive program, and calls for a high level of employee involvement and commitment to be effective. The use of PPE requires the choice of the appropriate equipment to reduce the hazard and the development of supporting programs such as training, change-out schedules, and medical assessment if needed.

1. Continue to use SCBAs when responding to vehicle fires. The fire fighters should don the SCBAs when they arrive at the scene and doff SCBAs only after overhaul is complete. This protocol should become written policy.

RECOMMENDATIONS
(CONTINUED)

Administrative Controls

Administrative controls are management-dictated work practices and policies to reduce or prevent exposures to workplace hazards. The effectiveness of administrative changes in work practices for controlling workplace hazards is dependent on management commitment and employee acceptance. Regular monitoring and reinforcement are necessary to ensure that control policies and procedures are not circumvented in the name of convenience or production.

1. Continue to position the motor pump operator and fire apparatus upwind of the vehicle fires to minimize exposures to the vehicle fire emissions.

2. Position the motor pump operator in an area upwind of the diesel exhaust from the fire apparatus. Diesel exhaust also contains hazardous substances.

REFERENCES

ACGIH [2009]. Threshold limit values for chemical substances and physical agents and biological exposure indices. Cincinnati, OH: American Conference of Governmental Industrial Hygienists.

Ahrens M [2004]. U.S. vehicle fire trends and patterns. Quincy, MA: Fire Analysis and Research Division. National Fire Protection Association.

Austin CC, Dussault G, Ecobichon DJ [2001]. Municipal firefighter exposure groups, time spent at fires and use of self-contained-breathing-apparatus. Am J Ind Med 40(6):683–692.

CFR. Code of Federal Regulations. Washington, DC: U.S. Government Printing Office, Office of the Federal Register.

Chan-Yeung M, Lam S [1986]. Occupational asthma. Am Rev Respir Dis 133(4):686–703.

EPA [1999]. Compendium Method TO-15, Determination of volatile organic compounds (VOCs) in air collected in specially-prepared canisters and analyzed by gas chromatography/mass spectrometry (GC/MS). In: Compendium of methods for the determination of toxic organic compounds in ambient air.

Cincinnati, OH: Center for Environmental Research Information, Office of Research and Development, U.S. Environmental Protection Agency (EPA) Publication No. EPA/625/R-96/010b [http://www.epa.gov/ttnamtil/files/ambient/airtox/to-15.pdf].

Evans D, Ku B, Birch M, Dunn K [in press]. Aerosol characterization during carbon nanofiber production: mobile direct-reading sampling. Ann Occup Hyg.

HSE [1999]. EH 40/98, occupational exposure limits 199.8. Sudbury, England: Health and Safety Executive (HSE) Books.

IARC [1982a]. Monographs on the evaluation of the carcinogenic risks to humans: some industrial chemicals and dyestuffs. Vol. 29. Lyon, France: World Health Organization, International Agency for Research on Cancer [http://monographs.iarc.fr./ENG/ Monographs/vol29/volume29.pdf].

IARC [1982b]. Monographs on the evaluation of the carcinogenic risks to humans: some industrial chemicals and dyestuffs. Vol. 29. Lyon, France: World Health Organization, International Agency for Research on Cancer [http://monographs.iarc.fr./ENG/ Monographs/vol29/volume29.pdf].

IARC [1983]. Monographs on the evaluation of the carcinogenic risks to humans: polynuclear aromatic compounds, part 1, chemical, environmental and experimental data. Vol. 32. Lyon, France: World Health Organization, International Agency for Research on Cancer [http://monographs.iarc.fr./ENG/ Monographs/vol32/volume 32.pdf].

IARC [1987]. Monographs on the evaluation of the carcinogenic risks to humans: overall evaluations of carcinogenicity: an updating of IARC monographs volumes 1 to 42. Suppl. 7. Lyon, France: World Health Organization, International Agency for Research on Cancer [http://monographs.iarc fr./ENG/Monographs/suppl7/ suppl7.pdf].

IARC [2006]. Monographs on the evaluation of the carcinogenic risks to humans: formaldehyde, 2-butoxyethanol and 1-tert-butoxypropan-2-ol. Vol. 88. Lyon, France: World Health Organization, International Agency for Research on Cancer [http://monographs.iarc.fr./ENG/Monographs/vol88/volume88. pdf].

References
(CONTINUED)

IPCS (WHO/International Programme on Chemical Safety) [2004]. International Chemical Safety card: formaldehyde [http://www.cdc.gov/niosh/ipcsneng/neng0023.html].

IPCS (WHO/International Programme on Chemical Safety) [2007]. International Chemical Safety card: carbon monoxide [http://www.cdc.gov/niosh/ipcsneng/neng0023.html].

Mabilia R, Cecinato A, Guerriero E, Possanzini M [2006]. Uncertainties of polynuclear aromatic hydrocarbon and carbonyl measurements in heavy-duty diesel emission. J Sep Sci 29(2):302–307.

Marand A, Karlsson D, Dalene M, Skarping G [2005]. Solvent-free sampling with di-n-butylamine for monitoring of isocyanates in air. J Environ Monit 7(4):335–343.

NIOSH [2005]. NIOSH pocket guide to chemical hazards. Barsen ME, ed. Cincinnati, OH: U.S. Department of Health and Human Services, Centers for Disease Control and Prevention, National Institute for Occupational Safety and Health (NIOSH) Publication No. 2005-149.

NIOSH [2010]. NIOSH manual of analytical methods. 4th ed. Schlecht PC, O'Connor PF, eds. Cincinnati, OH: U.S. Department of Health and Human Services, Centers for Disease Control and Prevention, National Institute for Occupational Safety and Health, DHHS (NIOSH) Publication No. 94-113 (August 1994); 1st Supplement Publication 96-135, 2nd Supplement Publication 98-119, 3rd Supplement Publication 2003-154. [http://www.cdc.gov/niosh/nmam].

Rugo H [2004]. Occupational cancer. In: LaDou J, ed. Current Occupational and Environmental Medicine. New York, NY: McGraw Hill Companies, Inc., pp. 229–267.

Siegmann K, Scherrer L, Siegmann HC [1999]. Physical and chemical properties of airborne nanoscale particles and how to measure the impact on human health. J Mol Struct-Theochem 458(1–2):191–201.

Smith D, Spanel P, Dabill D, Cocker J, Rajan B [2004]. On-line analysis of diesel engine exhaust gases by selected ion flow tube mass spectrometry. Rapid Commun Mass Spectrom 18(23):2830–2838.

REFERENCES
(CONTINUED)

Swedish National Board of Occupational Safety and Health [2000]. Occupational exposure values, Arbetarskyddsstyrelsens forfattningssamling, AFS 2000:3, Liber, Stockholm.

Ulfvarson U, Alexandersson R, Aringer L, Svensson E, Hedenstierna G, Hogstedt C, Holmberg B, Rosen G, Sorsa M [1987]. Effects of exposure to vehicle exhaust on health. Scand J Work Environ Health 13(6):505–512.

Volatile Organic Compounds

During the first evaluation, VOCs were sampled with evacuated stainless steel Summa canisters and TD tubes. The Summa canisters were used to collect 1 liter of gases and vapors from the vehicle fire emissions. The canisters under vacuum drew in 1 liter of air in less than 30 seconds. Particulate screens prevented particles from entering the canisters. The Summa canister samples were quantitatively analyzed for 75 VOCs out of 189 hazardous air pollutants listed in Title III of the Clean Air Act Amendments of 1990 [42 USC 85(i)(a)§7412] according to the EPA TO-15 Method [EPA 1999]. The TD tubes were used to sample air in the PBZs of the fire fighters. The TD tubes contained three beds of sorbent material: (1) 90 milligrams of Carbopack™ Y, (2) 115 mg of Carbopack B, and (3) 150 mg of Carboxen™. Aircheck 2000 pumps (SKC Incorporated, Eighty Four, Pennsylvania) were used for drawing airflows of 200 cc/min through the TD tubes. The samples were qualitatively analyzed for various VOCs according to NIOSH Method 2549 [NIOSH 2010].

Aromatic Hydrocarbons and Aldehydes

Calibrated SKC Aircheck 2000 pumps pulled 200 and 100 cc/min of air through the sampling media. Benzene, ethyl benzene, naphthalene, styrene, toluene, and xylenes were sampled with charcoal tubes (100 milligram/50 milligram) at a flow rate of 200 cc/min and analyzed with NIOSH Method 1501 [NIOSH 2010]. Formaldehyde and acrolein were sampled with XAD-2 tubes treated with 2-hydroxymethyl piperazine (120 milligram/60 milligram) at a flow rate of 100 cc/min and analyzed by NIOSH Method 2541 [NIOSH 2010]. However, to achieve better sensitivity, the XAD-2 tube samples were analyzed by gas chromatography equipped with a nitrogen phosphorous detector instead of the flame ionization detector as stated in NIOSH Method 2541.

Isocyanates

The sampling and analytical method used to measure isocyanates is described elsewhere [Marand et al. 2005]. The sampling media consisted of a denuder, a polypropylene tube (7 cm long, 0.8 cm diameter) attached to a 13 mm-polypropylene cassette. The inner wall of the tube was coated with DBA impregnated glass fiber filter (2.5 × 6 cm). The polypropylene cassette held a DBA impregnated glass fiber filter (13 mm diameter, 0.3 µm pore size). A calibrated SKC Aircheck 2000 pump was used to draw a flow rate of 200 cc/min through the tube and through the filter cassette. In theory, most gases, vapors, and aerosols are collected and derivatized in the filter cassette. However, MIC reacts too slowly with the reagent (DBA) to be collected solely with the filter cassette [Marand et al. 2005]. Thus, the primary purpose of the impregnated tube was to act as a denuder sampler for the low molecular weight monoisocyanates (e.g., MIC, EIC, ICA) and to enhance the derivatization efficiency by continuously replenishing the filter cassette with reagent [Marand et al. 2005]. The denuder samples were analyzed by the Institutet för Kemisk Analys Norden AB (Hässleholm, Sweden) under the direction of Dr. Gunnar Skarping according to the methodology described elsewhere [Marand et al. 2005].

Particles

Particles were sampled near fire fighters attacking fires using 25 feet of 4-inch diameter flexible aluminum ducting attached to a particle sampling platform described in detail elsewhere [Evans et al. 2010]. The sampling platform allowed simultaneous and continuous measurement of particles generated from fires in real time by multiple instruments. These instruments could not have otherwise been used close to the fires or the water spray from fire hoses. A blower unit downstream of the sampling platform drew contaminants or smoke resulting from the fires through the flexible ducting. Mean air velocities of between 1050 and 1300 ft/min were attained within the duct, resulting in contaminant residence times of approximately 1 second from duct inlet to instrument sampling probes. Sampling probes and inlets were selected and oriented to minimize particle sampling errors within the duct.

Particle concentration metrics included number, active surface area, respirable mass, photoelectric response and particle size distribution from 7 nm to 10 μm, provided respectively by a condensation particle counter (TSI 3007, Shoreview, Minnesota) with dilution, a diffusion charger (DC 2000CE, EcoChem Analytics, Murrieta, California), a photometer (TSI DustTrak™ 8520), a photoelectric aerosol sensor (PAS 2000CE, EcoChem Analytics, Murrieta, California), and an Electrical Low Pressure Impactor (ELPI, Dekati, Tampere, Finland). Air quality metrics (temperature, relative humidity, CO, and CO_2 concentrations) were also monitored from inside the duct (TSI Q-Trak™ Plus 8554).

References

EPA [1999]. Compendium Method TO-15, Determination of volatile organic compounds (VOCs) in air collected in specially-prepared canisters and analyzed by gas chromatography/mass spectrometry (GC/MS). In: Compendium of methods for the determination of toxic organic compounds in ambient air. Cincinnati, OH: Center for Environmental Research Information, Office of Research and Development, U.S. Environmental Protection Agency (EPA) Publication No. EPA/625/R-96/010b [http://www.epa.gov/ttnamitl/files/ambient/airtox/to-15.pdf].

Evans D, Ku B, Birch M, Dunn K [in press]. Aerosol characterization during carbon nanofiber production: mobile direct-reading sampling. Ann Occup Hyg.

Marand A, Karlsson D, Dalene M, Skarping G [2005]. Solvent-free sampling with di-n-butylamine for monitoring of isocyanates in air. J Environ Monit 7(4):335–343.

NIOSH [2010]. NIOSH manual of analytical methods. 4th ed. Schlecht PC, O'Connor PF, eds. Cincinnati, OH: U.S. Department of Health and Human Services, Centers for Disease Control and Prevention, National Institute for Occupational Safety and Health, DHHS (NIOSH) Publication No. 94-113 (August 1994); 1st Supplement Publication 96-135, 2nd Supplement Publication 98-119, 3rd Supplement Publication 2003-154. [http://www.cdc.gov/niosh/nmam].

According to a report by the U.S. Fire Administration [U.S. Fire Administration 2002], from 1996 to 1998, an average of 377,000 highway vehicle fires occurred, and nearly one quarter of all fire department responses during that time were to vehicle fires—more than the responses to residential property fires. Similarly, according to a report by the National Fire Protection Association [Ahrens 2004], in 2002, public fire departments responded to 329,500 vehicle fires, accounting for 20% of all reported fires, and since 1980, reported vehicle fires have fallen only 30%, compared to a 51% drop in reported structural fires and a 44% drop in fires of all types.

Despite the commonness of vehicle fires, only a few studies characterizing the emissions from vehicle fires have been reported in the literature [Wichmann et al. 1995; Lonnermark and Blomqvist 2006]. Most notable was a study by Lonnermark and Blomqvist [2006] where automobiles were burned in a controlled setting. Investigators in this study reported potentially harmful levels of hydrogen chloride, sulfur dioxide, aromatic hydrocarbons (benzene), PAHs, aldehydes (formaldehyde), dioxins and furans, and isocyanates. Many more studies investigating fire fighter exposures during structural fires have been conducted [Gold et al. 1978; Treitman et al. 1980; Brandt-Rauf et al. 1988; Jankovic et al. 1991; Bolstad-Johnson et al. 2000; Austin et al. 2001]. High levels (in excess of STELs) of CO, formaldehyde, acrolein, hydrogen chloride, hydrogren cyanide, sulphuric acid, and hydrogen fluoride have been reported during knockdown of structural fires [Jankovic et al. 1991]. Similarly, high levels of CO, formaldehyde, acrolein, glutaraldehyde, benzene, nitrogen dioxide, sulphur dioxide, and PAHs have been reported during overhaul of structural fires when SCBAs are commonly removed [Bolstad-Johnson et al. 2000].

From a particulate emissions perspective, little data have been reported in the literature to date. In the Lonnemark et al. [2006] vehicle fire study, particle size distribution measurements indicated significant submicrometer components for both particle number and mass. These findings suggest that the particulate component of vehicle fire emissions is of a size capable of reaching the gas exchange regions of lungs, where clearance mechanisms are least effective. Furthermore, PAHs were also indicated in both the vapor and particulate phases. These small particles may therefore provide a vector for not only depositing potential carcinogens, such as PAHs, into the deep lung tissues, but also onto the skin.

References

Ahrens M [2004]. U.S. vehicle fire trends and patterns. Quincy, MA: Fire Analysis and Research Division. National Fire Protection Association.

Austin CC, Wang D, Ecobichon DJ, Dussault G [2001]. Characterization of volatile organic compounds in smoke at municipal structural fires. J Toxicol Environ Health A 63(6):437–458.

Bolstad-Johnson DM, Burgess JL, Crutchfield CD, Storment S, Gerkin R, Wilson JR [2000]. Characterization of firefighter exposures during fire overhaul. AIHAJ 61(5):636–641.

Brandt-Rauf PW, Fallon LF, Jr., Tarantini T, Idema C, Andrews L [1988]. Health hazards of fire fighters: exposure assessment. Br J Ind Med 45(9):606–612.

Gold A, Burgess WA, Clougherty EV [1978]. Exposure of firefighters to toxic air contaminants. Am Ind Hyg Assoc J 39(7):534–539.

Jankovic J, Jones W, Burkhart J, Noonan G [1991]. Environmental study of firefighters. Ann Occup Hyg 35(6):581–602.

Lonnermark A, Blomqvist P [2006]. Emissions from an automobile fire. Chemosphere 62(7):1043–1056.

Treitman RD, Burgess WA, Gold A [1980]. Air contaminants encountered by firefighters. Am Ind Hyg Assoc J 41(11):796–802.

U.S. Fire Administration [2002]. Topical fire research series, vol. 2, issue 4: Highway vehicle fires. [http://www.usfa.fema.gov/nfdc/tfrs/htm].

Wichmann H, Lorenz W, Bahadir M [1995]. Release of PCDD/F and PAH during vehicle fires in traffic tunnels. Chemosphere 31(2):2755–2766.

Appendix C: Occupational Exposure Limits and Health Effects

In evaluating the hazards posed by workplace exposures, NIOSH investigators use both mandatory (legally enforceable) and recommended OELs for chemical, physical, and biological agents as a guide for making recommendations. OELs have been developed by Federal agencies and safety and health organizations to prevent the occurrence of adverse health effects from workplace exposures. Generally, OELs suggest levels of exposure that most employees may be exposed up to 10 hours per day, 40 hours per week for a working lifetime without experiencing adverse health effects. However, not all employees will be protected from adverse health effects even if their exposures are maintained below these levels. A small percentage may experience adverse health effects because of individual susceptibility, a preexisting medical condition, and/or a hypersensitivity (allergy). In addition, some hazardous substances may act in combination with other workplace exposures, the general environment, or with medications or personal habits of the employee to produce health effects even if the occupational exposures are controlled at the level set by the exposure limit. Also, some substances can be absorbed by direct contact with the skin and mucous membranes in addition to being inhaled, which contributes to the individual's overall exposure.

Most OELs are expressed as a TWA exposure. A TWA refers to the average exposure during a normal 8- to 10-hour workday. Some chemical substances and physical agents have recommended STEL or ceiling values where health effects are caused by exposures over a short period. Unless otherwise noted, the STEL is a 15-minute TWA exposure that should not be exceeded at any time during a workday, and the ceiling limit is an exposure that should not be exceeded at any time.

In the United States, OELs have been established by Federal agencies, professional organizations, state and local governments, and other entities. Some OELs are legally enforceable limits, while others are recommendations. The U.S. Department of Labor OSHA PELs (29 CFR 1910 [general industry]; 29 CFR 1926 [construction industry]; and 29 CFR 1917 [maritime industry]) are legal limits enforceable in workplaces covered under the Occupational Safety and Health Act. NIOSH RELs are recommendations based on a critical review of the scientific and technical information available on a given hazard and the adequacy of methods to identify and control the hazard. NIOSH RELs can be found in the NIOSH Pocket Guide to Chemical Hazards [NIOSH 2005]. NIOSH also recommends different types of risk management practices (e.g., engineering controls, safe work practices, employee education/training, personal protective equipment, and exposure and medical monitoring) to minimize the risk of exposure and adverse health effects from these hazards. Other OELs that are commonly used and cited in the United States include the TLVs recommended by ACGIH, a professional organization, and the WEELs recommended by the American Industrial Hygiene Association®, another professional organization. The TLVs and WEELs are developed by committee members of these associations from a review of the published, peer-reviewed literature. They are not consensus standards. ACGIH TLVs are considered voluntary exposure guidelines for use by industrial hygienists and others trained in this discipline "to assist in the control of health hazards" [ACGIH 2009]. WEELs have been established for some chemicals "when no other legal or authoritative limits exist" [AIHA 2009].

Outside the United States, OELs have been established by various agencies and organizations and include both legal and recommended limits. Since 2006, the Berufsgenossenschaftliches Institut für Arbeitsschutz (German Institute for Occupational Safety and Health) has maintained a database of international

OELs from European Union member states, Canada (Québec), Japan, Switzerland, and the United States available at http://www.dguv.de/bgia/en/gestis/limit_values/index.jsp. The database contains international limits for over 1250 hazardous substances and is updated annually.

Employers should understand that not all hazardous chemicals have specific OSHA PELs, and for some agents the legally enforceable and recommended limits may not reflect current health-based information. However, an employer is still required by OSHA to protect its employees from hazards even in the absence of a specific OSHA PEL. OSHA requires an employer to furnish employees a place of employment free from recognized hazards that cause or are likely to cause death or serious physical harm [Occupational Safety and Health Act of 1970 (Public Law 91–596, sec. 5(a)(1))]. Thus, NIOSH investigators encourage employers to make use of other OELs when making risk assessment and risk management decisions to best protect the health of their employees. NIOSH investigators also encourage the use of the traditional hierarchy of controls approach to eliminate or minimize identified workplace hazards. This includes, in order of preference, the use of: (1) substitution or elimination of the hazardous agent, (2) engineering controls (e.g , local exhaust ventilation, process enclosure, dilution ventilation), (3) administrative controls (e.g., limiting time of exposure, employee training, work practice changes, medical surveillance), and (4) personal protective equipment (e.g., respiratory protection, gloves, eye protection, hearing protection). Control banding, a qualitative risk assessment and risk management tool, is a complementary approach to protecting employee health that focuses resources on exposure controls by describing how a risk needs to be managed. Information on control banding is available at http://www.cdc.gov/niosh/topics/ctrlbanding/. This approach can be applied in situations where OELs have not been established or can be used to supplement the OELs, when available.

Vehicle Fires

Because vehicle fires are suppressed quickly (<15 minutes), STELs and ceiling limits should be used in determining safe levels of exposures. Tables 2 (on page 7) and 3 (on page 8) provide the STELs and ceiling limits for the chemicals we monitored in the PBZs of the fire fighters, except CO and acrylonitrile. The NIOSH ceiling limit for CO is 200 ppm [NIOSH 2005]. The NIOSH and OSHA ceiling limits for acrylonitrile are 22 mg/m^3 [NIOSH 2005]. The following section briefly summarizes the possible acute and chronic health effects from exposure to the compounds we sampled. Acute health effects from short-term exposures are the basis for most STELs and ceiling limits. However, because vehicle fires may account for up to 20% of all fire responses [Ahrens 2004], the potential chronic health effects from long-term or repeated exposures are also meaningful.

Aromatic Hydrocarbons

Short-term exposures to toluene can irritate the eyes and respiratory tract and may cause effects on the central nervous system; long-term or repeated exposures may also cause effects on the central nervous system, enhance hearing damage from noise exposure, and result in toxicity to human reproduction or development [IPCS 2002a]. Short-term exposures to naphthalene can cause effects on the blood, including lesions of blood cells (hemolysis); long-term or repeated exposures can result in chronic hemolytic anemia or cataracts [IPCS 2005]. Naphthalene is also considered possibly carcinogenic to humans [IARC 2002]. Short-term exposures to styrene may cause irritation to the eyes, skin, and respiratory tract, as well as effects on the central nervous system; long term exposures can defat the skin and also affect the central nervous system and enhance hearing damage from noise exposure [IPCS 2006]. Short-term exposures to xylenes may irritate the eyes and skin and affect the central nervous system; long-term exposures can defat the skin, affect the central nervous system, and may result in toxicity to human reproduction or development [IPCS 2002b]. Short-term exposures to benzene can cause irritation to the eyes, skin, and respiratory tract, as well as effects on the central nervous system; long-term exposures can defat the skin, affect the bone marrow and immune system, and lead to the development of leukemia [IPCS 2003]. Benzene is considered carcinogenic to humans [IARC 1982, 1987]. Unlike most STELs that are based on acute health effects, the ACGIH TLV STEL for benzene is based on the potential excess risk of leukemia from the dose rate-dependent toxicity of the compound [ACGIH 2001].

Acrylonitrile

Short-term exposures to acrylonitrile may cause irritation to the eyes, skin, and respiratory tract, as well as effects on the central nervous system; long-term exposures can have effects on the central nervous system and liver, and cause skin sensitization [IPCS 2001a]. Acrylonitrile is also considered possibly carcinogenic to humans [IARC 1999].

Aldehydes

Short-term exposures to formaldehyde can cause severe eye and respiratory tract irritation. Pulmonary edema is also possible. Long-term or repeated exposures to formaldehyde may cause cancer [IPCS 2004]. Formaldehyde is considered carcinogenic to humans [IARC 2006]. Acrolein is primarily an acute toxin. It is severely irritating to the eyes, skin, and respiratory tract. High levels of exposure can cause pulmonary edema [IPCS 2001b].

Isocyanates

Short-term exposures to isocyanates can cause irritation to the eyes, skin, and respiratory tract, and lead to asthma-like reactions, bronchitis, pneumonitis, and pulmonary edema [IPCS 1995]. Long-term or repeated exposures to isocyanates can cause respiratory sensitization and occupational asthma [Chan-Yeung and Lam 1986; IPCS 1995; ACGIH 2004]. Once sensitized, a worker can experience an asthmatic response from short-term exposures at levels below OELs [Chan-Yeung and Lam 1986; ACGIH 2004].

Carbon Monoxide

Short-term exposures to CO may affect the oxygen carrying capacity of the blood, resulting in asphyxiation and an increased risk for cardiac disorders. Long-term or repeated exposures can affect the cardiovascular system, central nervous system, and possibly cause toxicity to human reproduction or development [IPCS 2007].

Particles

Mechanistic understanding of the health effects of fine particulate matter on the human respiratory and cardiovascular systems is still in its infancy. However, numerous epidemiologic studies over the last few decades have consistently shown strong associations between elevations in ambient fine particulate matter concentrations and increases in short-term hospital admissions (morbidity) and mortality rates in the general population [Dockery et al. 1993; Seaton et al. 1995; Pope and Dockery 2006]. Those with pre-existing cardiovascular or respiratory disease, such as the young and elderly, are at greatest risk for adverse health outcomes.

References

ACGIH [2001]. Benzene. In: Documentation of the threshold limit values and biological exposure indices. Cincinnati, OH: American Conference of Governmental Industrial Hygienists.

ACGIH [2004]. Toluene-2,4 or 2,6-diisocyanate (or as a mixture). In: Documentation of the threshold limit values and biological exposure indices. Cincinnati, OH: American Conference of Governmental Industrial Hygienists.

ACGIH [2009]. 2009 TLVs® and BEIs®: threshold limit values for chemical substances and physical agents and biological exposure indices. Cincinnati, OH: American Conference of Governmental Industrial Hygienists.

Ahrens M [2004]. U.S. vehicle fire trends and patterns. Quincy, MA: Fire Analysis and Research Division. National Fire Protection Association.

AIHA [2009]. AIHA 2009 Emergency response planning guidelines (ERPG) and workplace environmental exposure levels (WEEL) handbook. Fairfax, VA: American Industrial Hygiene Association.

CFR. Code of Federal Regulations. Washington, DC: U.S. Government Printing Office, Office of the Federal Register.

Chan-Yeung M, Lam S [1986]. Occupational asthma. Am Rev Respir Dis 133(4):686–703.

Dockery DW, Pope CA 3rd, Xu X, Spengler JD, Ware JH, Fay ME, Ferris BG, Jr., Speizer FE [1993]. An association between air pollution and mortality in six U.S. cities. N Engl J Med 329(24):1753–1759.

IARC [1982]. Monographs on the evaluation of the carcinogenic risks to humans: some industrial chemicals and dyestuffs. Vol. 29. Lyon, France: World Health Organization, International Agency for Research on Cancer [http://monographs.iarc.fr/ENG/Monographs/vol29/volume29.pdf].

IARC [1987]. Monographs on the evaluation of the carcinogenic risks to humans: overall evaluations of carcinogenicity: an updating of IARC monographs volumes 1 to 42. Suppl. 7. Lyon, France: World Health Agency for Research on Cancer [http://monographs.iarc.fr/ENG/Monographs/suppl7/suppl7.pdf].

IARC [1999]. Monographs on the evaluation of the carcinogenic risks to humans: re-evaluation of some organic chemicals, hydrazine, and hydrogen peroxide. Vol. 71. Lyon, France: World Health Organization, International Agency for Research on Cancer [http://monographs.iarc.fr/ENG/Monographs/vol82/mono82-8.pdf].

IARC [2002]. Monographs on the evaluation of the carcinogenic risks to humans: naphthalene. Vol. 82. Lyon, France: World Health Organization, International Agency for Research on Cancer [http://monographs.iarc.fr/ENG/Monographs/vol82/mono82-8.pdf].

IARC [2006]. Monographs on the evaluation of the carcinogenic risks to humans: formaldehyde, 2-butoxyethanol and 1-tert-butoxypropan-2-ol. Vol. 88. Lyon, France: World Health Organization, International Agency for Research on Cancer [http://monographs.iarc.fr/ENG/Monographs/vol88/volume88.pdf].

IPCS (WHO/International Programme on Chemical Safety) [1995]. International Chemical Safety card: 2,4-toluene diisocyanate [http://www.cdc.gov/niosh/ipcsneng/neng0339.html].

IPCS (WHO/International Programme on Chemical Safety) [2001a]. International Chemical Safety card: acrylonitrile [http://www.cdc.gov/niosh/ipcsneng/neng0092 html].

IPCS (WHO/International Programme on Chemical Safety) [2001b]. International Chemical Safety card: acrolein [http://www.cdc.gov/niosh/ipcsneng/neng0090.html].

IPCS (WHO/International Programme on Chemical Safety) [2002a]. International Chemical Safety card: toluene [http://www.cdc.gov/niosh/ipcsneng/neng0078.html].

IPCS (WHO/International Programme on Chemical Safety) [2002b]. International Chemical Safety card: m-xylene [http://www.cdc.gov/niosh/ipcsneng/neng0085.html].

IPCS (WHO/International Programme on Chemical Safety) [2003]. International Chemical Safety card: benzene [http://www.cdc.gov/niosh/ipcsneng/neng0015.html].

IPCS (WHO/International Programme on Chemical Safety) [2004]. International Chemical Safety card: formaldehyde [http://www.cdc.gov/niosh/ipcsneng/neng0275.html].

IPCS (WHO/International Programme on Chemical Safety) [2005]. International Chemical Safety card: naphthalene [http://www.cdc.gov/niosh/ipcsneng/neng0667.html].

IPCS (WHO/International Programme on Chemical Safety) [2006]. International Chemical Safety card: styrene [http://www.cdc.gov/niosh/ipcsneng/neng0073.html].

IPCS (WHO/International Programme on Chemical Safety) [2007]. International Chemical Safety card: carbon monoxide [http://www.cdc.gov/niosh/ipcsneng/neng0023.html].

NIOSH [2005]. NIOSH pocket guide to chemical hazards. Barsen ME, ed. Cincinnati, OH: U.S. Department of Health and Human Services, Centers for Disease Control and Prevention, National Institute for Occupational Safety and Health (NIOSH) Publication No. 2005-149.

Pope CA 3rd, Dockery DW [2006]. Health effects of fine particulate air pollution: lines that connect. J Air Waste Manag Assoc 56(6):709–742.

Seaton A, MacNee W, Donaldson K, Godden D [1995]. Particulate air pollution and acute health effects. Lancet 345(8943):176–178.

Table D1. Ordered list of the 15 most abundant volatile organic compounds measured in the engine fire smoke with Summa canisters during the first evaluation

Order	Startup	Conc. (mg/m³)	Knockdown	Conc. (mg/m³)	Overhaul	Conc. (mg/m³)
1	Benzene	5.2	Toluene	9.3	Dichlorodifluromethane	48
2	Dichlorodifluromethane	5.1	m,p-Xylenes	6.2	Benzene	11
3	Propene	3.3	1,2,4-Trimethyl benzene	4.2	Propene	11
4	1,3-Butadiene	2.3	Styrene	3.3	1,3-Butadiene	4.8
5	Naphthalene	1.4	o-Xylene	2.9	Acetone	3.8
6	Toluene	1.4	Dichlorodifluromethane	2.4	Toluene	3.8
7	Styrene	0.83	Ethyl benzene	2.2	Styrene	1.6
8	Acrolein	0.56	Benzene	1.6	Acrolein	1.4
9	Methyl methacrylate	0.44	1,3,5-Trimethyl benzene	1.4	Chloromethane	1.2
10	Acetone	0.40	4-Ethyltoluene	1.4	Naphthalene	1.2
11	Ethanol	0.40	n-Hexane	1.1	1,2-Dichloroethane	1.1
12	Chloromethane	0.33	Propene	0.91	m,p-Xylenes	0.97
13	Acrylonitrile	0.32	n-Heptane	0.87	Acrylonitrile	0.77
14	Acetonitrile	0.28	Acetone	0.84	Acetonitrile	0.70
15	m,p-Xylenes	0.25	Ethanol	0.72	Ethanol	0.67

Table D2. Ordered list of the 15 most abundant volatile organic compounds measured in the cabin fire smoke with Summa canisters during the first evaluation

Order	Startup	Conc. (mg/m³)	Knockdown	Conc. (mg/m³)	Overhaul	Conc. (mg/m³)
1	Benzene	60	Toluene	4.6	Toluene	0.95
2	Acrylonitrile	27	Styrene	2.3	Styrene	0.45
3	Propene	18	m,p-Xylenes	2	Benzene	0.38
4	Acrolein	15	Acetone	1.9	m,p-Xylenes	0.33
5	Acetonitrile	14	n-Hexane	1.5	n-Hexane	0.31
6	Styrene	14	Benzene	1.4	Acetone	0.3
7	Acetone	12	Propene	1.4	n-Heptane	0.18
8	Chloromethane	11	n-Heptane	0.84	Naphthalene	0.17
9	Naphthalene	10	Methyl methacrylate	0.81	Propene	0.16
10	Toluene	10	o-Xylene	0.72	1,2-Dichloroethane	0.14
11	1,3-Butadiene	6.8	1,2,4-Trimethyl benzene	0.70	o-Xylene	0.12
12	Vinyl chloride	3.7	Ethyl benzene	0.70	Ethyl benzene	0.12
13	Vinyl acetate	1.5	1,2-Dichloroethane	0.67	Acrylonitrile	0.07
14	Ethyl benzene	1.4	Acrylonitrile	0.38	1,3-Butadiene	0.05
15	2-Butanone	1.1	1,3-Butadiene	0.25	Chloromethane	0.05

Table D3. Area air sampling results*

Fire	Sample location	Benzene (mg/m³)	Toluene (mg/m³)	MIC (µg/m³)	TDI (µg/m³)	ICA (µg/m³)	TRIG (µg/m³)
1	West	(0.11)	(0.07)	ND	ND	14.8	14.5
1	South	ND	3.68	ND	ND	6	5.9
1	East	ND	ND	ND	ND	ND	ND
2	West	(0.06)	(0.10)	ND	ND	ND	ND
2	South	ND	ND	ND	ND	ND	ND
2	East	ND	ND	ND	ND	ND	ND
3	West	(0.21)	(0.16)	8.8	3	60.2	66.8
3	South	ND	ND	ND	ND	ND	ND
3	East	ND	ND	ND	ND	ND	ND
MDC†		0.07	0.06	N/A	N/A	N/A	N/A
MQC		0.24	0.51	1.2	0.6	6.0	5.8

* Values in parentheses represent concentrations above the MDC but below the MQC.
† The analytical laboratory that analyzed the isocyanate samples did not provide an MDC or report values below the MQC.

Table D4. Summary of weather conditions during vehicle fire suppressions for the second evaluation

Wind	Vehicle fire 1 (75°F, 34% RH*)		Vehicle fire 2 (78°F, 31% RH)		Vehicle fire 3 (79°F, 33% RH)	
	Minutes at wind direction	Average wind speed (mph)	Minutes at wind direction	Average wind speed (mph)	Minutes at wind direction	Average wind speed (mph)
Southeast	8	3.6	2	2.7	0	N/A
South	6	2.9	1	3.3	11	1.7
Southwest	2	3.1	3	2.4	3	1.2
West	1	2.1	8	3.0	1	1.7
Northwest	0	N/A	2	2.1	2	2.1
North	0	N/A	0	N/A	0	N/A
Northeast	1	3.3	0	N/A	0	N/A
East	2	3.1	2	1.9	0	N/A

* RH = relative humidity

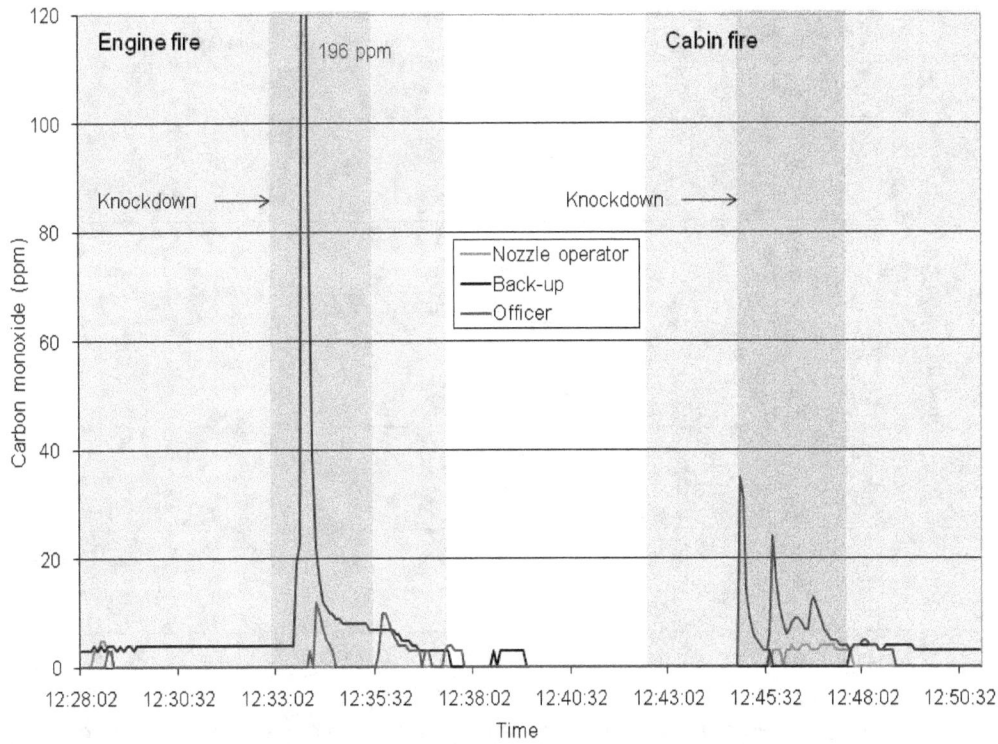

Figure E1. Personal breathing zone concentrations of CO during the first vehicle fire suppression on the second evaluation.

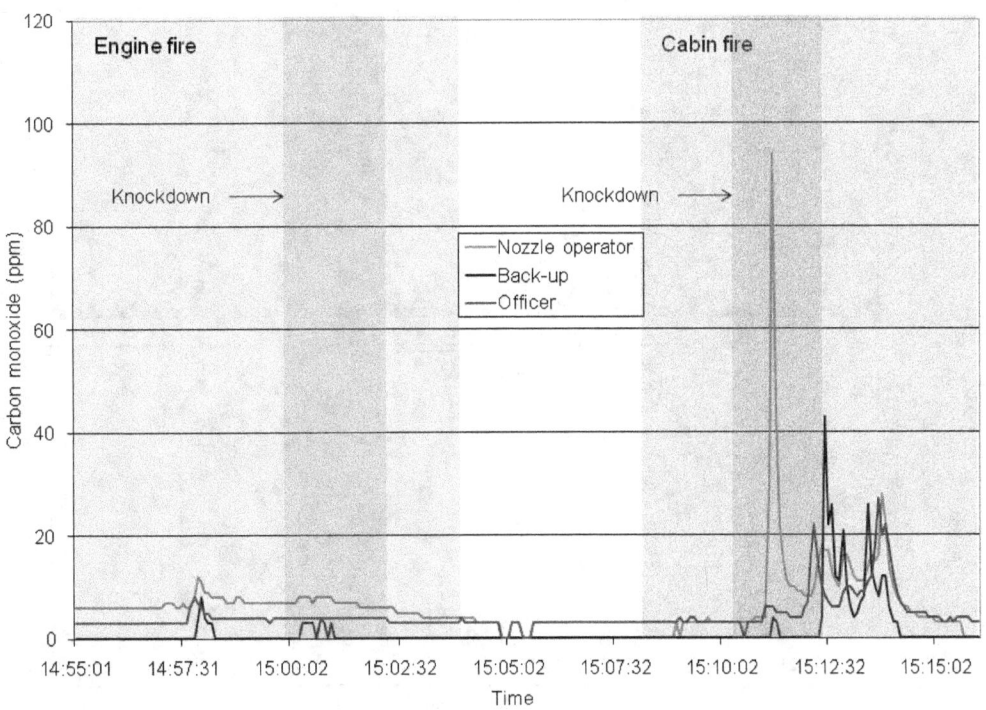

Figure E2. Personal breathing zone concentrations of CO during the second vehicle fire suppression on the second evaluation.

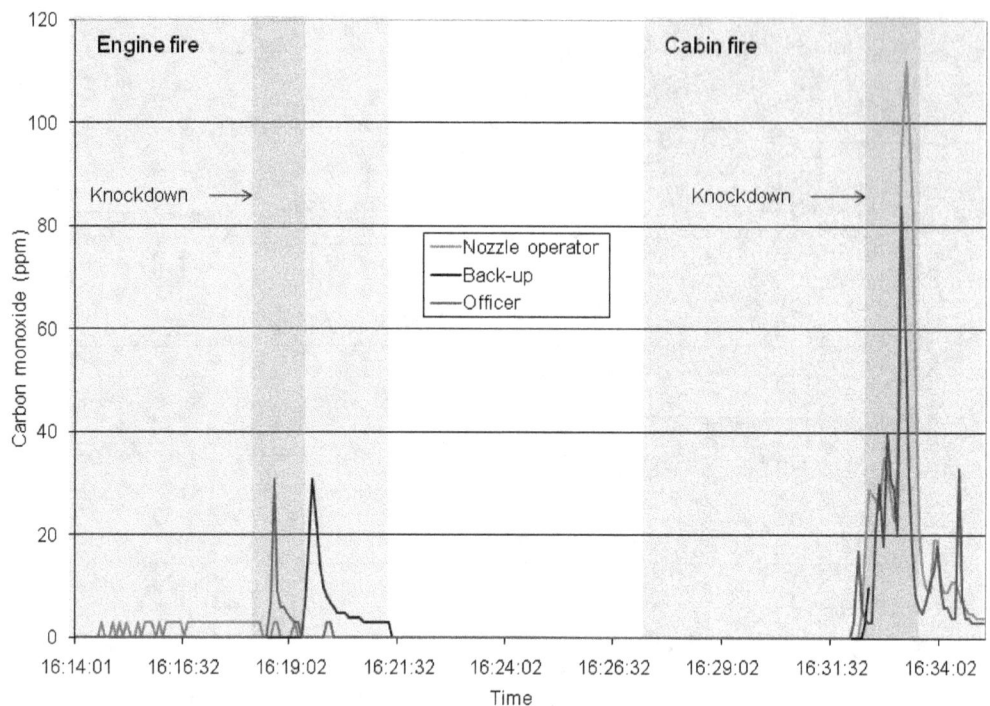

Figure E3. Personal breathing zone concentrations of CO during the third vehicle fire suppression on the second evaluation.

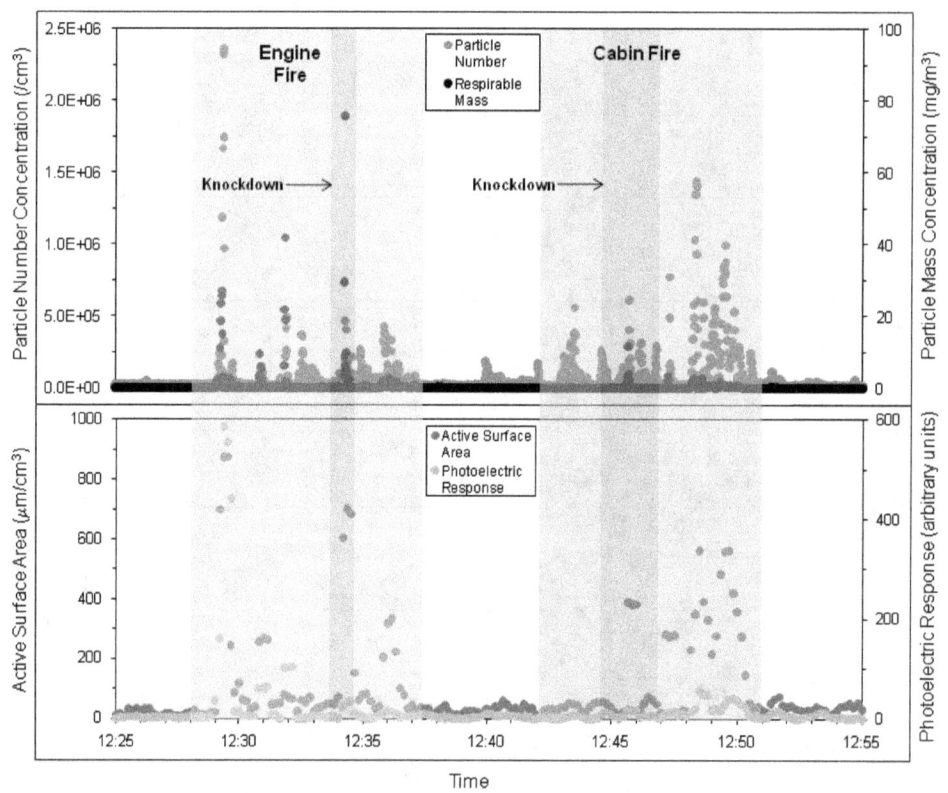

Figure E4. Particle measurements collected during the first vehicle fire suppression on the second evaluation.

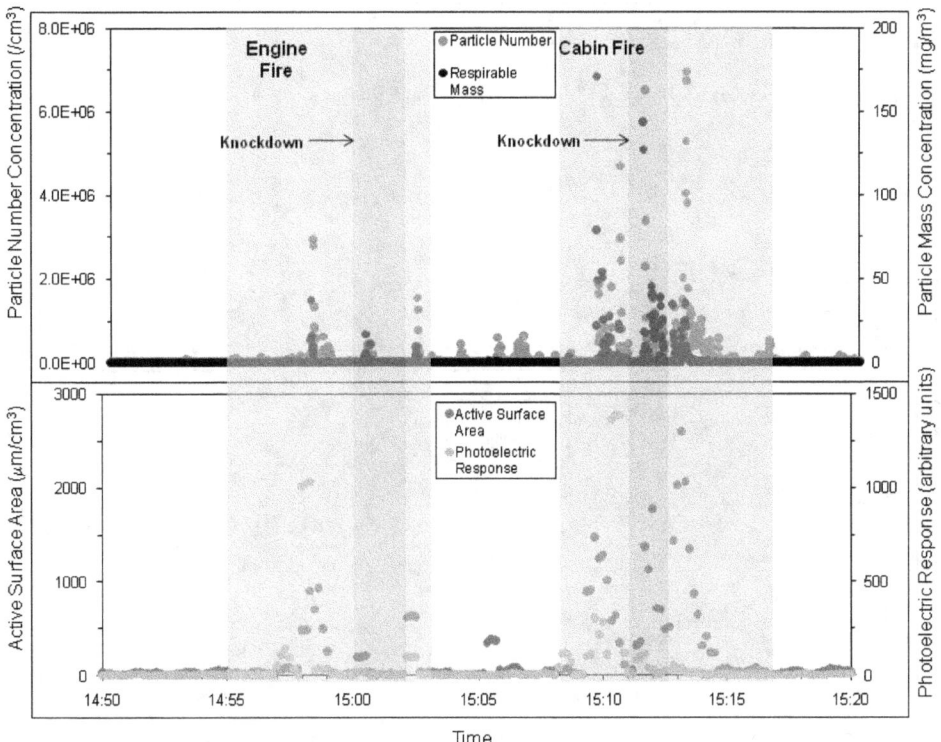

Figure E5. Particle measurements collected during the second vehicle fire suppression on the second evaluation.

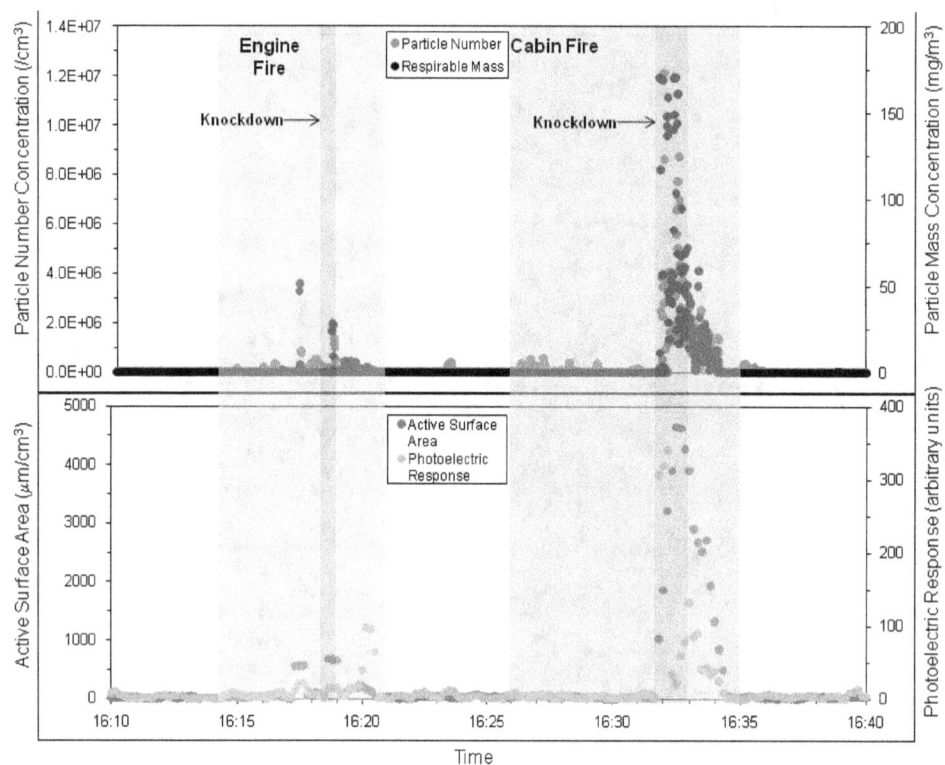

Figure E6. Particle measurements collected during the third vehicle fire suppression on the second evaluation.

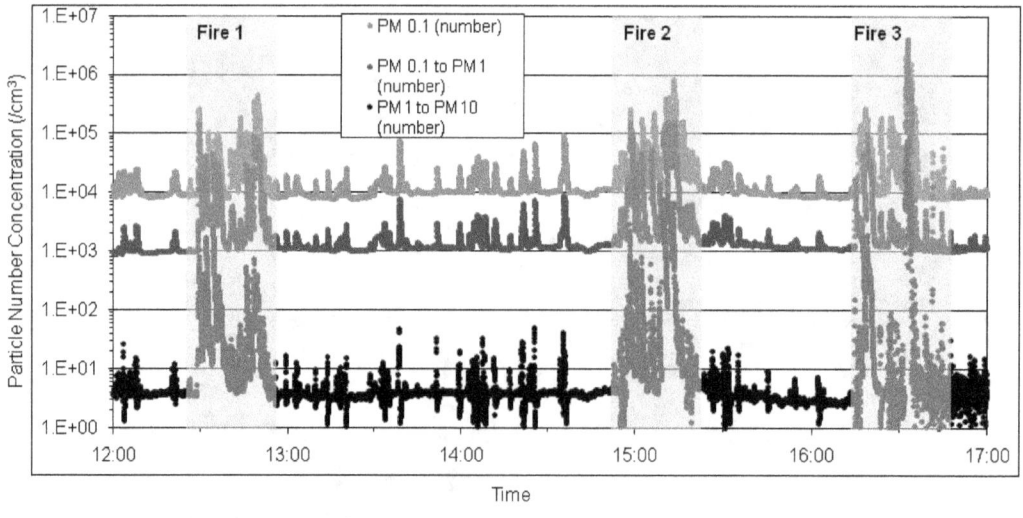

Figure E7. Particle number concentrations for different particle size ranges (< 0.1 μm, 0.1–1 μm, and 1–10 μm in diameter) throughout the day during the second evaluation.

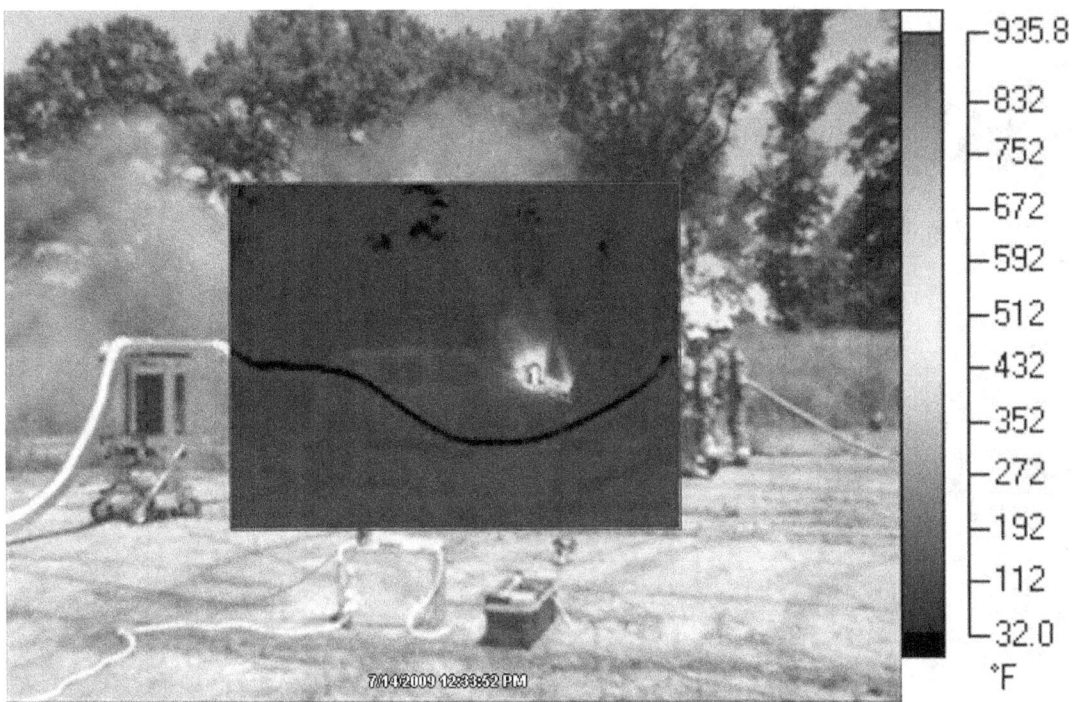

Figure E8. Thermal image of engine fire before knockdown.

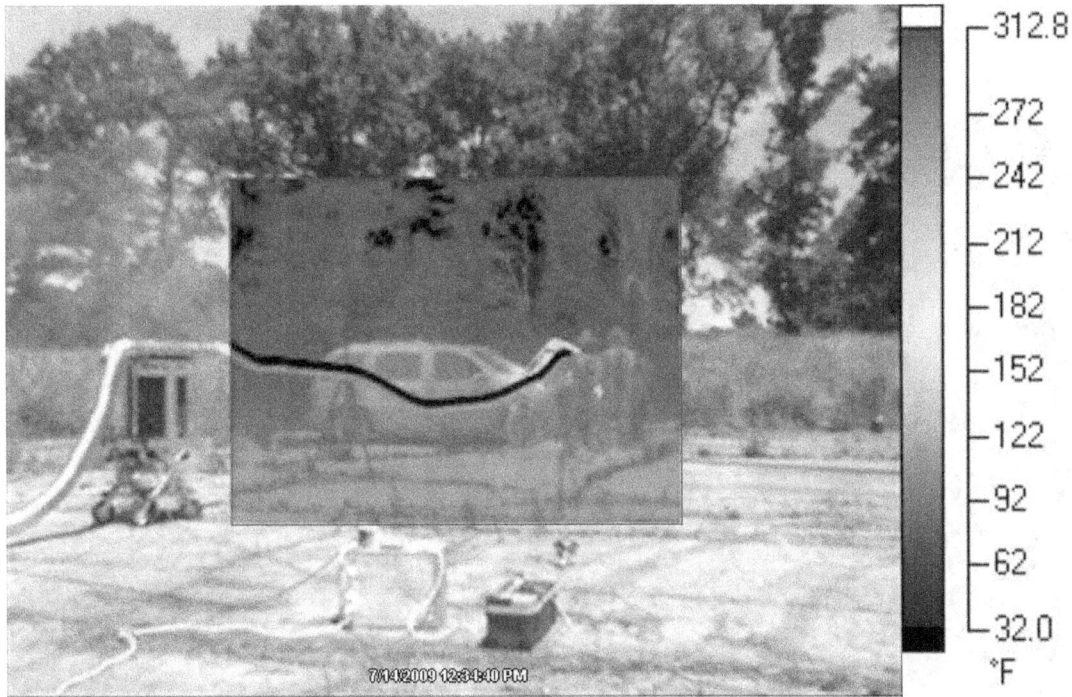

Figure E9. Thermal image of engine fire after knockdown.

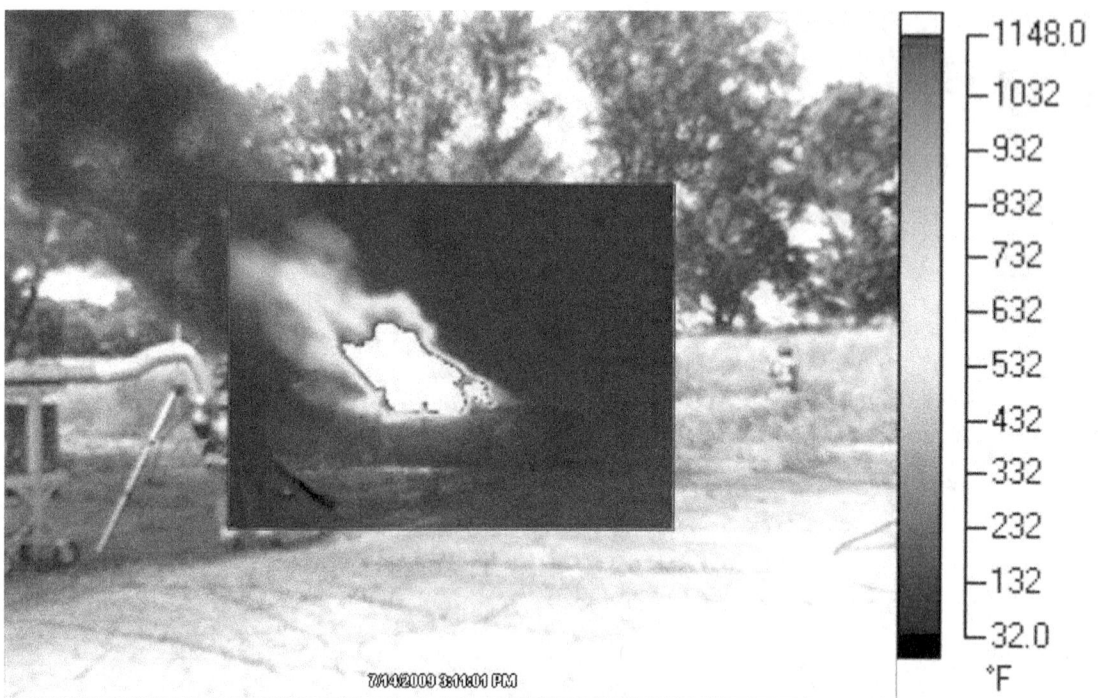

Figure E10. Thermal image of cabin fire before knockdown.

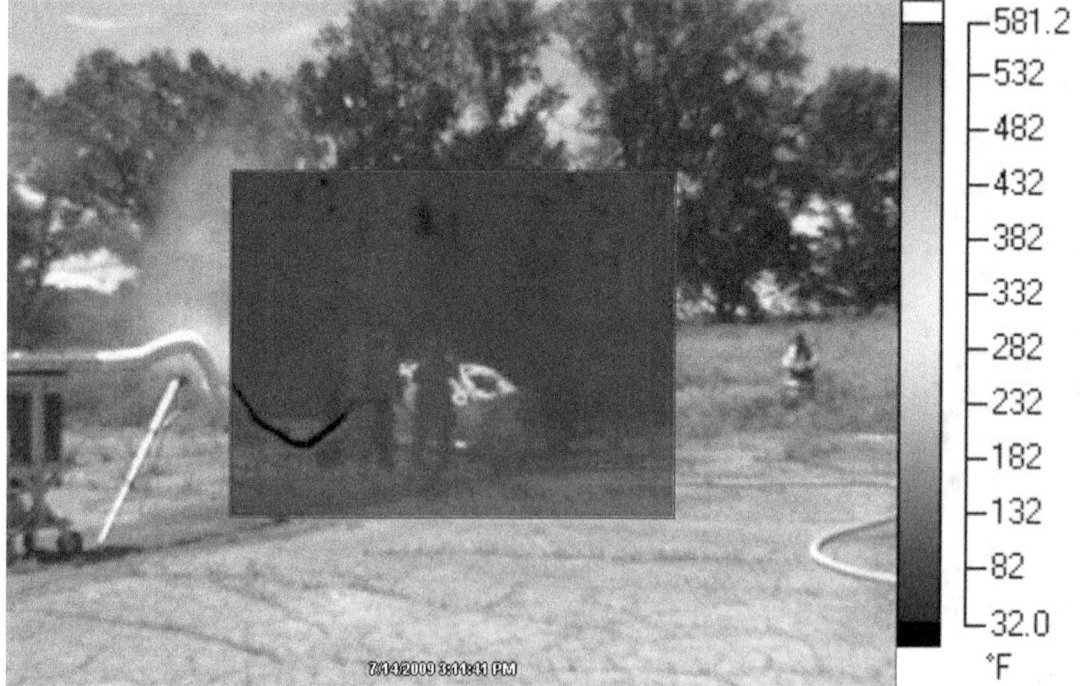

Figure E11. Thermal image of cabin fire after knockdown.

ACKNOWLEDGMENTS AND AVAILABILITY OF REPORT

The Hazard Evaluations and Technical Assistance Branch (HETAB) of the National Institute for Occupational Safety and Health (NIOSH) conducts field investigations of possible health hazards in the workplace. These investigations are conducted under the authority of Section 20(a)(6) of the Occupational Safety and Health (OSHA) Act of 1970, 29 U.S.C. 669(a)(6) which authorizes the Secretary of Health and Human Services, following a written request from any employer or authorized representative of employees, to determine whether any substance normally found in the place of employment has potentially toxic effects in such concentrations as used or found. HETAB also provides, upon request, technical and consultative assistance to federal, state, and local agencies; labor; industry; and other groups or individuals to control occupational health hazards and to prevent related trauma and disease.

The findings and conclusions in this report are those of the authors and do not necessarily represent the views of NIOSH. Mention of any company or product does not constitute endorsement by NIOSH. In addition, citations to websites external to NIOSH do not constitute NIOSH endorsement of the sponsoring organizations or their programs or products. Furthermore, NIOSH is not responsible for the content of these websites. All Web addresses referenced in this document were accessible as of the publication date.

This report was prepared by Kenneth W. Fent and James Couch of HETAB, Division of Surveillance, Hazard Evaluations and Field Studies (DSHEFS) and Douglas E. Evans of Engineering and Physical Hazards Branch, Division of Applied Research and Technology (DART). Industrial hygiene field assistance was provided by Manny Rodriguez, Chad Dowell, and Donnie Booher of DSHEFS. Photography assistance was provided by Fariba Nourian of DART. Videography was provided by Charles Urban of the Office of the Director. Analytical support was provided by Gunnar Skarping and colleagues at the Institutet för Kemisk Analys Norden AB, Bureau Veritas North America, and Columbia Analytical Services. Health communication assistance was provided by Stefanie Evans of DSHEFS and Amanda Harney of the Office of the Director. Editorial assistance was provided by Ellen Galloway and desktop publishing was performed by Robin Smith of DSHEFS.

ACKNOWLEDGMENTS AND AVAILABILITY OF REPORT

(CONTINUED)

Copies of this report have been sent to employee and management representatives at the Miami Township Fire and Rescue in Yellow Springs, Ohio, the Ohio Department of Health, and the OSHA Regional Office. This report is not copyrighted and may be freely reproduced. The report may be viewed and printed at http://www.cdc.gov/niosh/hhe/. Copies may be purchased from the National Technical Information Service (NTIS) at 5825 Port Royal Road, Springfield, Virginia 22161.

This page intentionally left blank.

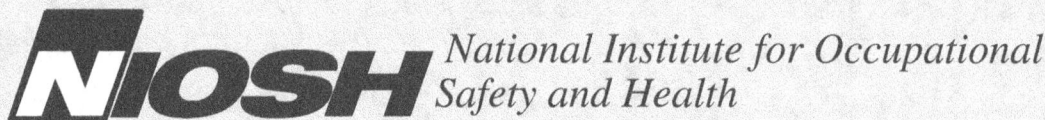

National Institute for Occupational Safety and Health

Delivering on the Nation's promise: Safety and health at work for all people through research and prevention.

To receive NIOSH documents or information about occupational safety and health topics, contact NIOSH at:

1-800-CDC-INFO (1-800-232-4636)

TTY: 1-888-232-6348

E-mail: cdcinfo@cdc.gov

or visit the NIOSH web site at: **www.cdc.gov/niosh.**

For a monthly update on news at NIOSH, subscribe to NIOSH eNews by visiting **www.cdc.gov/niosh/eNews.**

SAFER • HEALTHIER • PEOPLE™